ONLY
A LITTLE TIME

A Memoir of My Wife

ONLY
A LITTLE TIME

A Memoir of My Wife

by Sidney L. Werkman

Little, Brown and Company—Boston—Toronto

FIRST EDITION

T10/72

Library of Congress Cataloging in Publication Data

Werkman, Sidney L
  Only a little time.

  1. Leukemia--Personal narratives. 2. Werkman,
Alexandra Colt, 1939-1967. I. Title.
RC643.W47   616.1'55'00924 [B]   72-5131
ISBN 0-316-93090-3

Published simultaneously in Canada
by Little, Brown & Company (Canada) Limited

PRINTED IN THE UNITED STATES OF AMERICA

For Russell
May this guide you on your way

Preface

 For several weeks before the christening of our baby son in the early autumn of 1966, my wife, Alexandra, struggled with a sniffle and a feeling of tiredness that overcame her in the cool Washington evenings. During that season we often played tennis before dinner at the St. Alban's School or at the court of a friend. Several times, when dressing to play, putting on her socks or bending down to tie her tennis shoes, Alexandra, or "Sandy" as she was called, glanced at her lovely, sleek legs and asked, "Why do I keep banging my knees and getting these black-and-blue marks that don't go away? . . . And I wake up in a pool of sweat every morning?"

I bantered with her about these troubles, and though I made a doctor's appointment for her, I was not worried, for she was playing excellent tennis and kept up her usual schedule of teaching, caring for our son Russell, and arranging all sorts of happy activities for us to do together.

Then events of a single afternoon in October plunged us into dependence upon doctors and priests, the farther reaches of the human spirit, and a search of the deepest canyons and trenches of love and invention we possessed.

Those brief events ended in her death.

One moment she was a beguilingly fresh young girl and mother, waiting for my return each evening from Children's Hospital in Washington where I was a staff psychiatrist, reveling in a life unfolding happily with all the preparation of Boston, Cape Cod, boarding school, college, and Peace Corps work in Washington and Africa as a base. The next moment she was under a brutal sentence of death.

One brief look at a little drop of her blood placed under a microscope in her physician's office showed me that her illness was final, inexorable, hopeless. At that moment I had to learn about a new world and a different consciousness.

I had known that other world of terror and death at second hand from patients, but I was simply unprepared to explore it with my wife. Our happiness and marriage and long future dreams included no point of contact with death.

As I tell this story of a young and lovely woman, whom I adored far more than life, I must share intensely personal experiences and thoughts, for I cannot write about love without exposing both pride and pain, and I cannot approach agony without trusting a reader to be compassionate and even, at times, tolerant.

Because I am a physician, we could call on the friendly interest as well as the professional competence of other physicians; but I believe readers will recognize the pain and utter perplexity and occasional grandeur I try to describe as merely part of the common possibility and heritage we all share. I hope no reader will be offended by my attempts to search myself or by my pride in my wife. Though she was a unique woman I know that many other brilliant beings have wrestled gallantly with pain and death. I salute them and all who will follow in their path. But I write about Sandy in the hope that I may, somehow, reach out to those others and, through doing so, repay something of the gift her life was to me.

Sandy's death astonished me and leaves me bewildered still; but I have begun to understand, beyond the importance of our life together, the effect she had on other people, and both the emptiness and the legacy she has left in her passing. So, this is an account of love and pain during the last months of one human being — not famous or great, as the world weighs fame and greatness — whose life mattered because she could share delight and master harshness in turn, and help others to peer, however faintly, beyond calamity.

It is a book about noble physicians and nurses and medical students and pharmacists, for all of them combined to offer an interweaving of humane medical care that elevated the profession of medicine to its priestly origins.

I hope this story will give some direction and security to sick people, even ones traveling toward death, for having walked that path now, I can speak a bit about its roughness and its diversions. What I learned unfortunately couldn't be found in books — though I devoured a lot of writing about people dying — but from decisions made hastily and intuitively with Sandy as the pilot. As some people can, she drew out the finest qualities and sentiments of everyone caring for her. Once when I marveled to her physician about how sensitive and kind everyone in medicine had been with her, he answered, "Yes, but you don't see many like Sandy. It was what she was that brought it all out.

It's a two-way street. She gave as much to us as we gave to her."

The lives of those few unusual patients must be recorded as maps to guide the rest of us.

Finally, because Sandy received distinguished care throughout her illness, this is a book of thanks as well as a cautionary tale to all of us who are caretakers of other lives.

ONLY
A LITTLE TIME
A Memoir of My Wife

Chapter 1

 In a gray and often rainy Washington October, the sidewalks and streets of Georgetown yellow with a cover of fallen leaves, we prepared for our baby's christening. Friends brought over extra dishes and tablecloths. Grandparents arrived from Boston, an aunt and uncle from New York. We phoned in a large order for red wine and champagne to the liquor store.

Though unable to shake an "autumn cold," Sandy raced over to the florist in her little red Fiat convertible to choose flowers, to the French market to order a veal roast laced with kidneys, then back to our house in the "little red car." She was resolute in keeping the top of the convertible closed, for she was well aware of the attention she drew when driving with the top down, and, though

3

somewhat uncertain about whether or not she wanted to attract whistles from truck cabs high above her on the streets, her innate modesty swayed her decision. Tiredness forced her to take afternoon naps, and she told me plaintively, "I only weigh a hundred and fourteen pounds. I haven't weighed so little since I was a child. And why am I so bedraggled all the time? It's just not like me."

"I'll make an appointment for you with Buddy," I said, hoping to placate her. "It's probably just a flu bug. Lots of people have it now." As a physician myself, I had little concern about Sandy's mild symptoms, and arranged for her to see my cousin, Dr. Milton "Buddy" Gusack, an excellent internist, who, I was certain, would simply reassure her about her cold.

After Russell's christening and the happy lunch party on Sunday we waited, desultorily, for the appointment with Buddy on Wednesday. Relatives went off; a truck came to collect the rented chairs and the extra glasses needed for the christening party; tablecloths were returned; empty wine bottles were tossed in the trash. Sandy had a tea for some Opera Society people on Monday after teaching French at Potomac School in the morn-

ing. But her appointment book records Tuesday as
simply: "Bad day in bed."

Wednesday morning I gave an early lecture on
child psychiatry at the George Washington Medical School and then saw patients in my office at
Children's Hospital. My journal, written late that
sleepless night, tells the rest of the story:

Darling Sandy has had a "cold" with fever and tiredness this week. Because she began to have night sweats
and woke up in the morning drenched, my worst fear
was that she had tuberculosis. She went to see Buddy
Gusack today. I was confident nothing would be
revealed and without any real concern, for none of my
relatives or friends had ever had tuberculosis. It is an
old-fashioned illness.

We spoke about the opening opera on Friday, the
parties before and after it, and our hope to take Russell
and drive out to visit friends in Virginia on the weekend. I asked if Buddy had been gentle with her, trying
to get some more information, for I was surprised that
he had prescribed Achromycin, a potent antibiotic, for a
simple flu.

Sandy protested. "You told me he could be my doctor, and you are not meant to ask lots of questions about
a private relationship!"

I agreed with her and went on with the day at the
hospital. At 1:45 P.M. Buddy called me and said simply,
"Sandy has a lot of blast cells in her peripheral smear.
It's a leukemoid smear."

5

"What is her white count?" I asked.

"It's 12,000 and her hemoglobin is 10."

"Are you sure they're blasts?"

"Yes, and there are a hell of a lot of them."

"But she just called me and said you told her it was a flu bug and that I should pick up some Achromycin at Morgan's." I was bewildered and talking to try to get my scattered thoughts organized.

"I did, but that was before I saw the slide. I spoke with Arnold Lear and Ed Adelson about it and showed them the slide. There's no doubt. She'll have to have a marrow done in the morning. It may just be a leukemoid reaction to her infection, but if it isn't, we'll have to start treatment immediately. Tell her not to take the Achromycin."

I drove to Buddy's office and we talked and looked at the awful slide. And then I went home to Sandy, instructed to talk about the need for a bone marrow aspiration and nothing else. She was to be told "for the time being" that she had an anemia. "Dear God, may it be an anemia."

Sandy was tired tonight, but as sweet and softly loving to Russell and me as always. We went to bed at eight, but I came down here at ten, anxious and unable to sleep, though torn by the wish to keep holding her slight body and fevered wet hair in my arms forever.

"Dear God, make this illness a sign, a signal, and not a finality. Make it a leukemoid reaction to her cold.

"She is simply too pure of spirit, too good and decent and in need of comforting and sweetness, to have such an illness as leukemia course through her. She, if anyone in this world, doesn't deserve pain or the fear of death.

"She did so much for this great christening weekend. She gave it, as she gives everything she does, an atmosphere of ingenuous happiness that overwhelmed me and everyone else.

"I will be loving and accepting, and never curt or selfishly ambitious. I will cherish my life with Sandy and Russell and always be thankful for her. A brilliant career, more medical work in Asia, ability to write well — no desire I can think of begins to compare to my wish for her. I want Sandy healthy, Sandy at tennis, Sandy swimming, Sandy kissing our son — Sandy happy. Amen."

(When I wrote that entry, Sandy's physician, Milton Gusack, and I both knew she had leukemia, a deadly blood disease, and not just an anemia, a decrease in the number of red blood cells, or a leukemoid reaction, a moderate overproduction of white blood cells that sometimes accompanies infections. But a part of me still hoped for a miracle, even though the presence of great numbers of immature and nonfunctional white cells — myeloblasts, or "blasts" in medical jargon — in the peripheral bloodstream was an almost unmistakable sign of leukemia.

The other studies Dr. Gusack described, a white blood cell increase to 12,000, which is often seen in minor infections, and a hemoglobin level of 10 grams, suggesting the presence of a mild anemia, were of no real diagnostic importance. The crucial test still to be done was a bone marrow aspiration, the insertion of a hollow needle through the skin and into the middle of the breastbone in order to withdraw cells from the blood factory of the bone marrow, for the marrow is the key to diagnosis and treatment in leukemia. Those cells are then studied under a microscope to see if they are mainly the "blasts" Dr. Gusack had discussed with me.

It is the choking overproduction of white blood cells that characterizes leukemia, and the presence of overwhelming numbers of abnormal, immature white blood cells, "blasts," in the bone marrow factory that is a sure sign of the type of leukemia most resistant to treatment and most rapidly fatal — acute granulocytic or acute myeloblastic leukemia. In order to establish absolutely the type of leukemia Sandy had, it was necessary to see what the blood elements in the bone marrow looked like. That is why Dr. Gusack held out some tiny bit of hope to me on Wednesday.)

Slipping back into bed again I could feel her challis nightgown, now moist with fever, and her hair curled in little wet ringlets. I kissed her cheek and caressed her arm turned toward me. As I lay in bed, knowing that my wife sleeping next to me was filled with death, my thoughts scattered wildly. What preparation had there been for anything like this? What in the world is death?

It is the seventeen patients I pronounced dead when I was an intern. Images of some of them floated before me, particularly a little boy at the New York Hospital with nephrotic syndrome, a kidney disease. He always sat like a Buddha because of his grotesquely enlarged belly, looked into space, sometimes brushed back his little cowlick of hair, and waited. I considered it a great triumph to engage him in playing with blocks or a miniature shell game. But he did more and more staring, his little body increasingly filled with poison and death.

Sandy, as always, slept softly, and for the most part, comfortably. Occasionally in her dreams she called out in a muffled voice, "Russellino has to be fed. . . . Is he asleep? . . . I hear Russell crying. . . . Don't let him get hurt."

But she fell back into deeper sleep and dawn came.

Chapter 2

 Sandy's appointment book for Thursday merely records:

Buddy: 1:00 P.M.

Mrs. Lyons here: Teatime.

At dinner on Wednesday evening I told Sandy about the need for a bone marrow aspiration to discover what particular kind of anemia she had. I assured her that Dr. Rheingold, who was to do the procedure, had done thousands of them and that they were not painful. I told her that even I had done a number of them and that, surprisingly, the patients had lived.

Before going to bed I had said, "Darling, I'll drive you down and wait for you."

Sandy's answer was characteristic. "Well, if it isn't much, just a test, there's no need for you to stay away from the hospital. I feel a lot better now, anyway."

We dropped the question but my thoughts shifted back to the talk with Buddy. One of his statements echoed in my mind. "Sidney, if this is an acute granulocytic leukemia, she may die in a few days. We have to do a marrow tomorrow to be sure of what it is."

"I can't tell her everything tonight," I said, and began to cry.

"We have to do a marrow," Buddy gently persisted. "Maybe it is something different. A few cases have lived ten years. There's a registry of them."

"How old were they?"

"Mostly older than Sandy. But we can't say anything until we see the marrow."

I offered to tell Sandy how serious her illness was but Buddy, in the strongest terms, counseled me not to.

"But we've shared everything else. I don't know what to do."

"Tell her we think it is an anemia and probably related to the flu. But we need to do the marrow to be sure of what it is. Don't frighten her."

Frighten her. Which would frighten her more,

the use of the dreadful word leukemia, and its greater meaning, that she was dead though continuing to arrange flowers for our house, kiss me a loving good-bye each morning as I left for the hospital, cuddle and feed and wipe and fascinate our baby — or holding back on the use of that word and saying, instead, that she had an anemia? Some day, I thought, that withholding would come back at me and make Sandy lose all confidence in anything I told her. And, what was even worse, she would lose trust in me and believe that I did not respect her own ability to wrestle with tragedy and death. And then could I live with myself?

Relying on my own experience, my training in medical school and after, I would have told her. I remember many serious discussions, launched with the gravity of a high school seminar on sex, about the dying patient and what he should be told. All the fine surgeons and internists and psychiatrists would tease the subject, tickle it a bit, and then pronounce, with more than a little self-satisfaction and a massive dose of cliché: "All in all, when everything is said and done, the patient should be told his situation so that he can put his affairs in order and make his peace with the world."

Old people and old animals sometimes are serene enough to put their affairs in order and make their peace when they know death has invaded them. But someone twenty-seven years old, a young mother of a baby son, just reaching out into the life she fitted so well — should she be told to put her affairs in order?

I couldn't think clearly anymore and, instead, lapsed into a reverie about Sandy.

She was not a gossip or a person who enjoyed raking over the past and its injustices. Her manner of thought was the opposite of that. She told anecdotes of happy, charming events — of the winter her seventy-two-year-old grandfather went to Hot Springs, Virginia, crippled with arthritis and was so renewed by the waters that he took up ice skating again. Sandy always ended the triumphant anecdote with, "And, he died doing a figure eight on the ice."

She repeated stories told her by her father about his childhood. A favorite one concerned the time he, as a little boy, developed typhoid fever on a ship steaming into the Bay of Istanbul. All the port was alerted and a nine-year-old boy in a sailor suit was carefully lowered in the arms of his nurse to a launch waiting to take him to the English doctor onshore.

But a few themes of anguish and uncertainty slipped through. When Sandy was eight or nine years old, another girl tricked her into leaping from a precariously high roof to the ground and Sandy, trustingly, jumped. Though she was not hurt seriously by the fall, Sandy never understood how another girl could have been so cruel. When she was involved in the Peace Corps in Washington, working late over coffee, one of her bosses bent down and kissed her as he brought some manuscript for her to type. He then asked her out to supper. "I liked him a lot, but he was married, and it wouldn't go anyplace. Besides, I knew and liked his wife. He never looked me directly in the eye again," she said. But she told the story with a bit of longing and some poignance. And I think she added the part about "he never looked me directly in the eye again" for dramatic effect and, maybe, for my comfort.

Hospitals were her greatest fear. That isn't surprising, for, if you ask any patient, twenty-year-old or sixty-year-old, what he remembers of his childhood, a nightmarish hospitalization usually lurks in the background, a time of shadowy nurses, doctors poking around every part of the body, together with a panicky feeling of isolation, wondering what will be cut out next and if one's parents will ever come.

When she was seven, Sandy had a tonsillectomy

at the Children's Hospital in Boston. Her father promised her he would take her home in three days. She remembered that time in the words and fears of a child.

"They took off all my clothes and wrapped me in a sheet that was only big enough for a teddy bear and hardly covered anything. Then, there was a terrible doctor who made me open my mouth and move my arms, and he hurt me when he punched into my stomach. My real doctor, the one who took out my tonsils, was gentle and Daddy knew him. But this other one, he had a kind of Scandinavian accent, wasn't. He was the one who told me I couldn't go home on Thursday because I still had some bleeding in my throat. I told him my father said he would come and get me, but the doctor gruffly said he wouldn't. I cried and cried, partly because he was so mean and partly because my father didn't come until Saturday. It was horrible."

She was such an open, innocent creature, so direct and, I thought, vulnerable. A fusion of beguiling adult and naïve, trusting child characterized every moment in her friendships, teaching and committee work, loving, and caring for Russell.

Another medical incident illustrated this fusion of child and adult in her clearly. Before we were married Sandy stayed home from the Peace Corps one day, aching and feverish. I broke off my work at Children's Hospital and went to her house to see her in the midafternoon. She was lying in bed wearing a challis nightgown that reached down to her toes. Her hair, which had a tendency to curl when damp, was moist with heat and parts of it were plastered against her forehead. She looked very young and, though sick, she tried to be both intimate, for we knew each other very well, and formal, for I was there to examine her and see what should be done. Both of us were uncomfortable and a bit excited.

I had my doctor's bag beside me. After examining her head and eyes and inside her mouth, I asked to lift up her nightgown so I could palpate her abdomen. She shook her finger at me mischievously, but drew down the covers to let me reach under her nightgown. I assured her of my medical seriousness as I poked at her left and right side. I listened to her chest with my stethoscope and then placed my hand over her heart, including a bit of her lovely small breast as I felt for her heartbeat.

After I finished my examination and told her what medicine to take for the flu, she drew me down on the bed, took me in her arms, and kissed me with no discomfort or embarrassment at all.

She was truly grateful that I had come immediately when she was worried, and in addition she was responding as a woman to our mutually felt excitement. The experience showed, in addition to how much we were drawn to each other, that she was not comfortable in having people touch her body medically. She was part grown-up, part child, not really certain that the doctor would find her well. Perhaps he would say she must stay in bed through Christmas vacation or that she would have to take an evil-tasting medicine.

Chapter 3

 On the afternoon of her test, as I recalled these memories, the physician in me, the lover, the person who identified with a beloved wife were hopelessly snarled. Fortunately, the conflict was ended by Buddy, wise Buddy.

"Don't tell her. I promise you it will be better not to tell her. I know, Sidney. I've watched people die the minute they're told. I've watched husbands and wives disintegrate. That's a lot of horseshit that people feel better if they're told. Maybe you, maybe some doctors, but not many. It's cruel."

After clearing the lump in my throat several times, I asked, "How can I live with it? How can I stand it?"

Buddy said, "You've got to."

And I went home to Sandy. I drove slowly back to our house from Buddy's office and put down my briefcase in the hall. I patted Niccolo, our West Highland White terrier, and looked at the Chinese painting flowing down from the steep staircase, swaying precariously as it always did. I knew I must go up that staircase to speak with Sandy, as Gloria, Russell's nurse, said she was in the baby's bedroom putting away diapers.

The room was our first bedroom in this tall, brick house. When Russell was moving energetically in his mother's abdomen, we decided to move our bed into another room next to this one, and make our bedroom into his nursery.

In this room we read, looked out the window at the great maple tree, and put up Russell's first mobile. In this room, also, Sandy wore her challis nightgowns to bed and was delighted to have me slip them off over her head so that our bodies could be close. She was utterly unselfconscious when she lifted up her arms before we held each other and made love. Because of shared love the room was filled with memories of great happiness and mischievous delight.

In this very room Russell might have been conceived. But he wasn't. We decided to begin him during a vacation at Cape Cod, before I had to go off to Afghanistan and Iran on a Peace Corps trip. So, instead of sailing or riding or playing tennis we spent a good many short afternoons close together, in the great Italian phrase, "making the miracle." And Russell was conceived there, for when I returned from Asia and we drove to Washington, Sandy knew that a baby was growing in her.

This bedroom in Washington, with its happy memories for Sandy and me, now held Russell's crib, his bassinet, a chaise longue, a little pine chest of drawers made in Pennsylvania in 1803 and several rickety wooden chairs, as well as a high-backed white rocking chair.

The whole future of our life together was molded by the events of that cool Wednesday evening in October as I walked up the steep steps to the second floor of our house, bewildered and with no heart for life. I turned the corner, opened the door into the nursery, and saw Sandy in a very short pale-blue silk kimono bending over Russell's bassinet putting away some diapers. As she bent down the lovely curve of the back of her long slim legs reminded me for a moment of happier thoughts. She straightened, turned, and welcomed me with a sparkling smile. Behind her face, the orange leaves on the large maple tree outside reflected sunlight through the window. Russell gurgled happily and raised himself up on the side of the crib. I went to her, realizing that I had not, finally, decided what to say or not to say. On the verge of crying, I took her in my arms and we kissed. I brushed my hand across the back of her hair, pulling her toward me in that brief moment when passion and reason intermingle, when everything in you wishes to obliterate the world and leave only the two of you. But Sandy interrupted what I wanted to be an eternity, with a question. "Did you get the medicine?"

Should I tell her? Should I tell her that I had seen the slide spelling her doom in Buddy's office, that I now understood what is said about drowning men, that all of their lives appear before them in the few seconds before breath leaves forever?

I cleared my throat. "Buddy called me after you spoke with him. He believes you have an important anemia, in fact, he thinks . . ." I couldn't continue. I just held her close to me.

Sandy waited expectantly an instant, then pulled my head to her shoulder and said, "Well, it doesn't matter so long as they know what to do about it. I don't care about taking pills and I'll do everything that they tell me to do. There's no need to cry. I'm sure it will be over in a month or so. And, darling, Russell is here and gurgling away, so don't talk about it anymore."

Did she minimize the awful message underlying Buddy's words to me? Was she afraid to hear more? Or did she sense the true meaning of my loss of control and react, not out of embarrassment or lack of concern, but from an elemental courage bred in her and nurtured by years of training, that allowed her to meet challenge directly and with a certain understated defiance? I think it was courage, a courage that sometimes may have seemed mere bravura or casualness, but, in fact, represented a formidable reserve of strength.

She wanted to hear no more about her "anemia," and I knew very well that I couldn't talk about it any further, that I would follow her lead, and that we had chosen a way of faith and hope and, probably, fantasy.

In later times when pain began or she was extremely weak and puzzled, and asked "Why does this keep on? I've always done everything I'm supposed to do and taken all of the pills, and it just doesn't help," I would try to explain a bit about blood disease and point out that recovery took a long, long time. Often, I was ready to begin a detailed, distorted description of her illness, but she

was always comforted by simple medical statements and really wanted to know very little more
about the physiology and pathology of anemias,
and of what the future might hold. She was easily
assured about life and needed very little support to
live in the moment. Any deeper thoughts remained
within her.

But Sandy was not unique. Most patients don't
want to know the meaning of a blood urea nitro-
gen test or listen to a detailed interpretation of the
ominous tracings of an electrocardiogram. They
want to know that you are responsible for them
and will care for them. Perhaps parents want to
know and need to hear diagnoses in the most definitive words possible, but not others.

I knew, and I felt helpless with the weight of my
knowledge. We are simply unprepared for the
death of people we love. Our own death, our own
wish to be out of pain or trouble, yes. But we don't
conceive our children and feed them and play with
them and watch them grow with any thought that
they will leave us in death. Neither do we hold
hands and become lovers, nor do we talk about
curtains and dishes and bassinets and the long future of summer vacations and winter accomplishments, with any thought that our lovers will leave
us.

On that afternoon a malignancy suddenly was implanted in me, and I had my own death to figure out, for her illness abruptly marked the end of the happy illusion of timeless existence. This realization was too much for me to encompass, especially with Sandy there with me, a bright example of everything meant by the word life.

Chapter 4

 What an example she was, "what a glorious creature," as one of our friends described her. Sandy was difficult to get all in focus, because the usual terms of definition — faults, roughnesses, oddities — had little application to her. She knew very little about pettiness, ridicule, cynicism, great jealousy or even irony.

Sandy's physical presence radiated health and energetic delight. She was tall, and her long, slim, active body fitted very well into pleated, plaid skirts and knee socks or short tennis shorts. She had soft, clear skin, the pristine skin of a child, sprinkled with freckles over her nose and eyes. Eager, smiling, brown eyes identified Sandy, particularly the modeling of her upper eyelids that slanted outward, giving her entire face a look of bewitching oddity, as if she were partly Tibetan or Chinese.

Her straight nose was singularly expressive, squinching up with pleasure and capable of expressing surprise, tentativeness, curiosity or humor, just as if it belonged to a most alert, superior forest animal.

She lived with form surrounding her. She delighted me and smoothed our weeks by planning regular Thursday evening dinner parties and Saturday lunches. She arranged tea visits with women of every age and knew that we would go to the museum on Sunday afternoon if we were not wheeling Russell around the brick sidewalks of Georgetown. And the year culminated in a Santa's workshop of Christmas cards, followed by the mailing, with real pleasure, of presents to each one of her many nieces, nephews and special friends.

From the beginning I viewed Sandy from a skewed vantage point. I adored her. First because she was so physically lovely; later because she had such startlingly ingenuous but magically beguiling ways; finally, because she came to love me and to impress a meaning on my life I had not known before.

She wrote letters assiduously to a legion of friends, old and young, in a thin, run-together scrawl, though the only ones I received date from a period before we were married when Sandy was in Paris working and studying music, and I was based in Italy writing a book. Several of these letters, which I include now, reflect some of the reasons I wanted to be with her whenever possible.

Darling Sidney,

My most uncreditable sleepiness was just wearing off properly when it was time to say good-bye this morning. So many things to say — but mostly I hope that the squeak from my partially hidden voice was loud enough to convey the complete joy at hearing you would be here Friday evening. It is so much the dream I have been dreaming. My heart has been singing all morning. (No idea of going back to sleep.) Thinking of this and what you might most enjoy doing — I did not listen very carefully to the explanation of how I should start my teaching job tonight, when I talked to my motorcy-cle-riding boss.

And as if to reflect the sun of Florence you spoke of, the Paris sun came out and lit the Seine and the Rue de Rivoli just as the bus crossed the river — dazzling.

The Saint-Simon can have us, though I am going to look into other possibilities — and all these lovely paintings and sculptures are at your command — as is your very loving

Alessandra

My Darling Sidney,

I am sitting in bed at a late hour — midnight — with the music of Berlioz in my ears. The "Damnation of Faust" I saw tonight was captivating to Paris critics and has been to audiences, too. I enjoyed it tremendously though it is a very unusual interpretation — a great deal of ballet, principally two dancers who take the parts of Faust and Marguerite and are particularly moving in their interpretation of the two souls' despairing, but ever-powerful love in hell.

It was my first time in the Paris Opera House and a thrill to see it. The singers, as you warned, were not inspiring, though Marguerite and the Devil were, at times, very good to my ear. I missed you more profoundly than ever — as I always feel particularly close to or lost without you when listening to music. I especially sought out and stood in the same spot in the Opera where you said you were thinking of me when you were here last alone.

Though it is still not warm, it is more spring than ever, and I walked all the way to the Musée d'Art Moderne along the Seine. I noticed new things — particularly details of the elaborate Pont Alexandre III. Do you remember its gold horses and, on the Right Bank, the charioteer and rearing horses on the side of the Grand Palais which are almost a part of the bridge? They are the same style. I remarked particularly among the many statuary on the bridge itself, a young girl with a shell to her ear. I will show you.

Today was so sunny. Paris was a dream — and one felt quite in a dream walking around. How I longed for you and wished your hand had been in mine. And that we had been together seeing the children playing with rubber balls in the Tuileries. (The balls kept getting lost under benches and the feet of snoozing men and it was amusing to watch the little elfs retrieve them!) Some music made by students drifted in — a very lingering, slow atmosphere.

I am so happy to be here in the spring for I see now the full charm of this fairy-queen city, a charm I have never felt before.

My lambie pie — I wish I could paint with bright strokes the walls of your house so your work will be similarly bright. I hope you are pleased with your writing but not so much that you do not think of Paris.

If you have time would you clarify something for me which I remember your saying? Was it that the definition of Opera is Tragedy?

Do all operas have to end tragically —

From reading these letters you may think she was simply one of nature's favored, carefree spirits. Though blessed in many ways, she did have certain problems. Large, formidable parties were an ordeal for her and she evaded them whenever possible or stayed close to my side and coaxed me to leave quickly when we had to go to one. At the start of our own parties she squeezed my palm tightly in her wet fingers, anxiously wiggling and turning her hand in mine as she made little comments when guests came in the door of our house.

"How lovely to see you."

"Wendy, your article on Italian food in the *Post* was delicious to read."

Neither of us was gifted with brilliant wit or quick conversation at odd moments, but I had been at it longer and could depend on words such as "marvelous" and "great" to cover long pauses. Sandy was more likely to talk about flowers and the Opera Society and how well children looked, though her ultimate refuge was the world of Boston and the Cape and all her relatives.

The night we met, at a small reading group, Sandy appeared wearing a short wool skirt that showed off the lovely curve of her legs as she sat back in her chair. A group of young CIA, World Bank, and lawyer friends, bored by Washington cocktail parties at which no topic could be discussed in any depth, decided to meet regularly and argue over the meaning of such dissimilar books as Camus's *The Stranger* and *The Divine Comedy*. Sandy joined us the evening we were puzzling over *The Last Puritan*. All the rest of us had read the book and were jousting over various interpretations of Oliver Alden's behavior. Sandy had little to say during the detailed discussion, but as everyone else let up a bit, she admitted, "I only got to read

the first few chapters, but I know the story because
Santayana wrote the book about my cousin."

All of us were taken aback and intrigued at the
same time by Sandy's ingenuous statement. She
went on to describe Harvard involvements and relatives around Boston. She warmed up to questions
about mutual relatives and friends and, for a few
minutes, we departed from all talk of *The Last Puritan*. And so it went for the rest of our lives together. I kidded her often after parties with statements such as "Darling, you never have to know
anything about anything except your family. As
soon as they hear about Cape Cod, all you have to
do is preside while people brag about the time they
came to Tarpaulin Cove or Hadley Harbor." She
would wag her finger at me in mock censure, but
was pleased by the attention she got.

During the first few months we knew each
other, we met casually at the reading group,
dances and other parties. Certainly she was a
lovely creature, but I found myself wondering
whether her guilelessness represented a beatific
simplicity or just the meandering of a pretty girl
who was saved from slipping into Bennett Junior
College by a fortunate late acceptance to Bryn
Mawr. And, I know she had no serious thoughts

about me, for, shortly after we met, she disconcerted me by saying that one of the reasons she was drawn to me was that she felt she could trust me to help her medically in case she ever got sick.

I think it never occurred to her that I would ever be anything more than an older friend, like the many pleasant bachelors in Washington who were regularly invited to large black-tie dinner parties and took out young things to expensive lunches at Rive Gauche, expecting nothing, except that the girls smiling brightly across the silver and flowers would listen appreciatively to their stories and jokes and help them feel more alive.

But I did hope for more, for I was not exactly in the mold of the black-tie bachelor. We continued to brush against each other at our reading group, Sunday lunch parties and dances, until everything changed, not by making love, but through the kind of magic that sometimes descends happily on the world to remind us of perfection.

Just before Christmas, I drove Sandy to the railroad station on her way to New York. As the car skidded uncertainly down K Street to the old Union Station on a snowy morning, I asked her casually if she would like to go out to dinner and a small dance on New Year's Eve. I prefaced all this with standard hypocritical disclaimers about how dull New Year's Eve was and how much above it we were. Sandy chimed in with the same tune, saying that she would be happy to come to dinner with me if she got back from New York in time. We agreed that New Year's Eve was a tiresome, overblown excuse for parties, tawdry and without the spontaneity that made some evenings such fun.

She did return in time and, after a Mexican dinner peppered with rather stiffly amusing talk about Boston and Europe, we drove to a party at a friend's house. Many friends were there standing in front of fireplaces to keep warm and waiting for midnight. Midnight came with its mildly pleasant excitement and I pecked Sandy a dutiful kiss on her closed lips, not really caring to do more. It was all amusing as we talked with other friends, crisscrossed each other in one room or another of the house, and ambled into the early moments of the New Year. As in a lazy game of bicycle tag we used to play late at night in a vast plaza on the island of Kos in Greece, Sandy and I gradually came closer and closer together. Then we found ourselves dancing in the basement, warmed by a leaping fire, alone. As we swirled around to a rock tune, my arms over her shoulders, her hands on my hips, our cheeks grazed and we drew closer. A kiss then transformed convenience and pleasantness, kindness and beauty to simple love, a love that made it important only to live or die for Sandy, to give anything, say anything, or leave everything unsaid for Sandy.

We left the party and walked silently through new-falling light snow that made all the world a hushed reflector to our misty breathing and sat, stunned, in my car under a lamp light for a happy eternity. The few kisses we shared were not especially passionate. They lingered endlessly, our lips brushing, not certain where to turn next.

And then, for the first time, I understood why the mystic Jews of the Old Testament groped for a name for the all-encompassing concept we call God — Yahweh, the ineffable, the unnameable. Love is God, total, eternal, beyond definition. It is the energy that infuses the happy saint who sells fruit from a truck, and the lack of love creates the ironies and sighs in the lives and acts of more famous figures. Francesca traced it all clearly when, under Paolo's tutelage, she turned from her reading of script one day, leaving a last line: *Quel giorno più non vi leggemmo avante* (That day we read no further).

On New Year's Day, I returned to Sandy's house at noon to pick her up and go to a lunch party in the country. As I drove toward the little place where Sandy and her roommate Jeannie lived, my head was still swimming with the delight we had shared in waking Jeannie at dawn, only a few hours earlier, and drinking a bottle of champagne to the New Year with her before kissing each other on the doorstep a last time.

A little handwritten note fluttered on the red door: "Have had to go out to lunch with Jeannie. Longtime invitation. Completely forgot. See you tonight at Robin's. Sandy"

With this note, discord came into our lives, repeatedly and with an agony that only mad lovers can devise. We saw each other, barely, at the evening dinner. Sandy appeared with Jeannie and left early with Jeannie, even though I phoned her saying I would pick her up, take her home, do anything. She was very pleasant, just as if I were a cocktail companion, chattering away for a few moments about nothing.

Sandy flew to Germany for the International Peace Corps; I went to Columbus, Ohio, to speak about adolescence; we met at parties. But the snow came and the February slush of Washington. At "The Dancing Class," a party held regularly in Washington, endless times we brushed against each other. I waited for the evenings of the reading group, where we read *Don Quixote, The Divine*

Comedy and then *The Adventures of Augie March*.
I scratched at Augie March in airports on the way
to Nepal and in a sickbed in Bangkok, naked electric light blinding me and a noisy air-conditioner
freezing my toes. The talk was desultory and
Sandy was at reading group meetings sometimes
and away sometimes. Never did she go home with
me.

One evening she agreed to go out to dinner. We
quickly ate some pasta at the Trieste on Pennsylvania Avenue, escaped through the tangle of beads
that guarded the front door, and went to a movie
across the street. Rita Tushingham swam her wide
eyes through a painful opus about a longshoreman,
a pregnancy and a lot of misery. I held Sandy's
hand, which became hot, slippery and elusive. The
hotter it got, the less connection there was between us. Her hand might just as well have been
severed at the wrist and allowed to rest in my palm
as a fried potato.

We spoke little as I drove her home. Finally, as I
turned the corner between Twenty-eighth Street
and the Oak Hill Cemetery, I stopped the car and
parked.

"Sandy, I just care so much for you, I can't let
things go on in this way," I told her.

Sandy said, too confidently, "I'm sorry but I just

don't have the same feelings. I like you, but I like a number of other men. I never expected we would get so close. I don't feel the same way. I think it would be best for us not to see each other this way anymore."

"What about New Year's and the other times?" I pleaded.

But she brushed further talk aside airily and asked that we drive to her house.

As I bent to switch on the ignition I turned to her and whispered the only words I could say. "You can choose not to see me, Sandy, but you can't stop me from loving you."

Sandy answered consolingly, "I think very highly of you, and I just wish it were different."

Talk trailed off and the lampposts of R Street, the Oak Hill Cemetery and Dumbarton Oaks Gardens slid by us before we turned down to Thirty-second Street and Sandy's house to say our good-nights.

I knew too well what separated us, or thought I did. I was eleven years older than Sandy and, in the tight compartmentalization of college and graduate school eras, had been formed by different friends, different experiences. Also, I carried with me a lifelong feeling of homelessness and uncertainty that I believed I could never share with anyone else.

Because I was by many years the youngest child in a family that, for many reasons, was running a different course from mine, my early experiences tied me warmly to a black nursemaid, not my mother, to loneliness and a wish to escape rather than appreciation for the virtues of honesty and uncomplaining hard work and decency that so surrounded me. I turned away when still very young from being a Jew and the son of Jews from Lithuania and Russia to explore a far different world from the one they knew, carrying with me a legacy of vulnerability that resonated between intelligence and arrogance, self-assurance and doubt. The legacy also included a love of music and a considerable introspective bent.

My father had had a short career as an operatic baritone before going into business, and I grudgingly admired and feared his impeccable musical taste, which formed a little island of purity in an otherwise broken and disdainful man. I followed his musical direction and became a serious clarinetist as a young boy but looked for something more. I found the beginning of what I was seeking on cold Sunday afternoons listening to organ recitals in the dark Episcopal Cathedral in Washington,

D.C., a twelve-year-old surrounded by widows and old men. That led me to a religion and community of solitude and privacy in contrast to what I saw as the prying, pigeonholing curiosity of Jewish families. When I began playing clarinet professionally in jazz bands as a young adolescent I learned quickly about champagne fountains, the insides of glittering houses, marijuana, laughing girls, steaming chafing dishes filled with scrambled eggs and bacon at midnight, the difference between the blue neon glare of ratty roadhouses and the soft light of the Sulgrave Club ballroom. I knew which light I preferred.

In the classic American immigrant tradition I became embarrassed by my parents because they seemed to talk only about inanities, troubles, food and their "successful" relatives, whom I hardly knew. I had not yet learned that there were far more corrosive faults than half-delighted envy of a relative who had become rich.

At the same time I stumbled onto that universal library cherished by a particular group of isolated young adolescents — *David Copperfield, Les Misérables, Arrowsmith, A Farewell to Arms, Islandia, The Great Gatsby, Of Human Bondage, The Possessed, Look Homeward, Angel*, and many more. Fortunately, I also read Sir William Osler's inspir-

ing book of essays about the profession of medicine, *Aequanimitas*, which probably saved me
from a life of moonstruck wandering. However, at
the time I believed more in Gatsby than in Sir William Osler, and passed quietly into the world of
country club tennis and strolling accordion players
at Long Island dinners, though I felt exceedingly
odd about the entire performance.

When Sandy and I were first together I wondered how I could have deserved her, whether I
was merely a pleasant visitor, tolerated by an un-
fathomable graciousness that might turn into rejec-
tion. But I felt that only partly, for I knew that I
had a certain intelligence and taste, a considerable
musical ability, a now built-in comfort in talking
with all kinds of people and a delight in pleasing
others that came from endless experiences in new
situations. And I had been fortunate in love before,
so, at least a part of me knew how little externals
mean to lovers.

Sandy's family frightened me. Boston families
are, indeed, different. They seem to inherit a
unique disease whose main symptom is rapture of
the profound, great past. This symptom helps
sufferers through endless dinner parties and visits
to every part of the world. The disease is similar to

gout, always a center of conversation, occasionally painful and crippling, but extremely convenient to explain away lack of present productivity, while hinting at great reserves of untapped ability. Other manifestations of the disease may be a refusal to speak of money or a paradoxical feeling of security that permits open discussion of odd deaths and suicides, desperate cousins hiding away in Somalia and all manner of events that turn others to blushing or psychoanalysis.

Sandy's background was not untainted by the disease. As she said of one of her relatives, "He peaked too young. He was at his best when he was captain of the hockey team and a prefect at boarding school. Somehow," she mused, rubbing her cheek during an unusual moment of philosophizing, "things never worked out as well for him afterward." When I found that the disease was not dangerous to others, I became a bit more comfortable in approaching her family.

Mr. Henry Colt, Sandy's father, had been a colonel in the United States Army during the Second World War. Since the war his chief apparent glories have been making excellent martinis, despite the use of sherry instead of vermouth, gamely fighting the catbrier on Cape Cod, and telling endless but precisely and charmingly articulated stories about "the War," Santa Barbara in 1932, his childhood, certain racehorses of many years past and his father's exploits in Turkey and Geneseo, New York.

"Now, Sidney, if I've told you this, stop me. Only a damn *fool* (and how he emphasized "fool") would repeat stories." And he would launch into, "When the war began (the First World War) a friend and I left school and reported to a shipyard, ready to work. Well, the foreman was astonished to see two fifteen-year-olds before him, but he said . . ." His heavy upper eyelids slanted and half-shut, long face partially scowling and a martini in his hand, off he would go. We would wait for the end of a story heard many times, then disperse to play pool.

Sandy grew up hearing her father's stories, seeing her mother in a long dress and her father in black tie for dinner every night except Sunday. Mrs. Colt, always darting about changing flowers and humming, moving like a young bird or a charming ingenue, totally open about her psychiatric hospitalization, turning to me at dinner to inquire about new research in mental illness, and then describing the visit of an Asian holy man who came to stay with her family at the seashore one summer, after living his entire life in the scorching heat of India, only to suffer a sunstroke on Cape Cod. Conversation flitted in that household, as Mr. Colt said so many times, "like a fly on the open pages of the encyclopedia." It was impossible to pursue any subject, no matter how important, around a corner, for another one was there ready to lead you astray.

When I wanted to marry Sandy, having no experience with asking a father for his daughter's hand, I tried to speak with him quietly about the seriousness of my intentions. I asked if he would join me in his small library. He trudged behind me, reluctantly, as if I were a school headmaster about to censure him for chewing gum in class. I began to expound on my love for his daughter and my resolve to be a good husband. Before I'd properly warmed to the subject, he jumped up from the trunk he was crouching on and leapt for the door, mumbling, "Humph, well. Now what was Andy Smith drinking? Could you go and ask him again?" He was just too uncomfortable to talk about such subjects, turning instead to charmingly impersonal, extended anecdotes and light ironies. I assumed he would be concerned about my financial status and Jewish family background, but he wasn't at all.

I harbored my own concerns about Sandy's family, even if they voiced none about me. Repeatedly, on speaking with people in New York or Washington about my coming marriage, I would be asked, "Who are her parents?" And I came to anticipate the deprecating response. "Oh, Harry Colt, poor Harry. He was absolutely the wittiest man in Boston, but what has happened to him? What has he done with himself?"

But such people as well as I at that time were unable to distinguish a relic from a sleeping giant. Mr. Colt was ready to wake and act at a moment of crisis, though on first glance he may have seemed merely a minor remnant from America's past.

Sandy and I compounded the problems of families and personal doubts with geographical ones that scattered one or the other of us on work assignments, at various times, to Paris, Germany, Singapore, the Ivory Coast of Africa, Florence, and Palm Springs, California, before we were married. We exhausted all the ways of escaping and coming together we could dream up and, though those ways had a fascination for us, they are not unknown to other lovers. Finally, we stumbled our way around all the barricades set up for each other, and our wedding day came and erased, literally, all the uncertainty of the past.

On the day we were married I gave Sandy a silver mirror with this quotation from Dante inscribed on its back: *Che siete angelicata criatura* (For thou art an angelic creature).

This angelic creature was now beyond help. All the landmarks and plans of a lifetime had to be compressed into a few days or a few months at most. Though I couldn't find a pattern then, I did feel that if Sandy and I allowed ourselves to drift, to glance at each other over breakfast every morning with death in our thoughts, the true malignancy would be a fascination with death itself. I searched desperately among the mixed claims of fate, chance, fear, closeness and hope for some direction that might obliterate the spell of death.

$Chapter$ 5

 I turned first to the church in the person of Les Glenn, an Episcopal minister I liked very much and who had spent summers at the same boys' camp on Lake Champlain I had attended. When Sandy was getting ready for bed, I slipped down to my study and called him, asking whether I could talk with him the next morning. Though I said it was important, I told him I could come some other day if it would be more convenient for him but he cut in with, "Of course, you can come tomorrow morning. Come and have a cup of coffee at seven-thirty."

At Les's house I was ushered into his sunlit library. Wearing a wrapper over his trousers, round white collar and black shirt, he offered me coffee. We spoke of Camp Dudley, where both of us had played music and appeared in original plays. I interrupted, needing to get directly to the point. "Les, Sandy has a very serious disease, leukemia."

He asked me for details, and I told him she might die in a few days. "It's called acute granulocytic leukemia, and I've been given no hope by her doctors, no hope at all for her." I described what leukemia was and why the particular form she had was so lethal. I became increasingly the effective physician, describing in layman's terms the details of an illness, I suppose trying to spare Les some of the pain that I had come to ask about. I suppose, too, that one of my reasons for coming to see him was the hope that some miracle might be possible. Though I scoffed at that thought, I still had a remnant, as many of us do, of the childish belief in faith, turning over a new leaf, being good and having God reach down and help. As I talked about medicine and little blood corpuscles, bone marrow, and the body being ravaged by disease, I lost my belief in immortality and became increasingly direct in my discussion and began to wonder why I had bothered Les. I became rather embarrassed about the whole idea of bothering him and turned to a different issue.

"All I want is some way of dealing with this." Then I began a trite sentence which brought on the most helpful and important statement of Sandy's entire illness.

"Les, I know we all have to die sometime . . ." I was going to continue and say that all I wanted was some way for me to be strong and helpful to Sandy during these last awful times.

Les cut in, "Why yes, we all do have to die sometime" — his voice trembled with its peculiar high, musical quality — "but for her, it should be forty years from now."

Neither of us said anything for a moment, but a miracle had occurred. In some way, that interchange gave me the help I needed. I had expected that Les would offer warmth, advice from his long experience about the awesomeness of death, and tell me ways of accepting and living with the life that was still present. He knew a lot about these things, in contrast to physicians, who keep people alive medically but have no concern about preparing them for death because death is a failure for medicine. But what he said, "For her, it should be forty years from now," had a mystically assuaging effect upon me, for it emphasized the absurdity of her situation.

We then discussed details of her illness and gradually returned to talk of the ordinary world. Les recalled how beautiful Sandy was and reminisced about the time he was minister of a church in Cambridge, Massachusetts, where her mother and father lived, and about what a handsome couple they were. He then went on to speak of faith and his belief that many people could overcome illness through faith. He knew an Episcopal minister in Washington who was still living, in fact living more effectively than ever, twenty years after a cancer of the colon had mysteriously regressed, apparently because of his faith. In his charming way, Les repeated, "Yes, faith is often better than anything. I'm sure that healing can occur through faith. I know that it can."

Here we parted company, but his belief was comforting to hear. The first five minutes of our talk had given me everything. I did ask him about things that Sandy and I might read, and he told me of two books, *A Diary of Readings* by John Baillie and Baron von Hügel's *Selected Letters*. Les took my hand in both of his and, as we parted, said, "I'll do anything for you. You know I'm available. Come back and see me soon, whenever you want. And give my love to your dear girl."

But all the last was unnecessary, for his one statement was incandescent and the readings and the books and the miracles were superfluous. Sometime later I told Sandy about the books and we got them. We read aloud sections from them in the morning, daily homilies on difficulty, faith, optimism and charity. But in truth, they bored us, for they didn't speak to our world and its finality.

From Les Glenn's house I went to Children's Hospital to see my own patients, wiping my eyes and clearing my throat on the way. Sandy had her bone marrow aspiration done.

Thursday was one of Washington's truly glorious days, with strong yellow-orange sunlight and coolness in the air as the leaves fluttered down in their clusters of autumn dampness. I finished seeing patients early and, with the connivance of my secretary, left the hospital around three in the afternoon because Sandy had called and said she wanted to play tennis. I would have happily climbed a mountain or chopped ten cords of wood to get rid of the tension, and readily agreed to tennis. In fact, I'm sure I encouraged the delusion that we could continue our life just as it always had been.

I came home to find Sandy in her tennis shirt and short white shorts, tying her tennis shoes. I quickly changed, gave Russell a hug, and we drove several blocks up Thirty-first Street to the Friendlys' tennis court. Jean and Alfred Friendly's tennis court was a gathering place for young and old, al-

ways in use and surrounded by friends of the
Friendlys playing bridge or reading the Sunday
New York Times as they waited to get on the court
for the next set.

While brushing fallen leaves from the court in
order to make it playable we had a short chat with
Mrs. Friendly, just as if Sandy were a usual Sandy.
We hit the ball back and forth about twenty minutes before she sighed, "Darling, I think that's
enough for now. I'm just too tired to play anymore." I knew it was a reckless thing we had done,
but it gave us both great delight, and we walked
off with our arms around each other's waists back
to the little red car, and drove home for tea.

That was the last time we ever played tennis.

Later, I drove down to Buddy's office to see the
marrow slides. We gathered in Buddy's office—
Buddy, Arnold Lear, Edward Adelson and Jack
Rheingold, all hematologists. A slide of Sandy's
bone marrow had been set up on the microscope.
We all looked learnedly at it, commented on its
symmetry, and said a lot of other foolish things.
But it was all show from here on. Arnold Lear was
going to take care of the hematological aspects and
Buddy the general medical needs. Buddy suggested we send the slide to Dr. Dameshek, a famous hematologist in New York, and to other

hematologists in Boston and at Johns Hopkins. He offered to take Sandy to Johns Hopkins on Saturday for a consultation in case I had any doubts about the diagnosis. It is remarkable how cool and professional we can remain under conditions of hopelessness. Naturally, I needed no confirmation, only treatment.

We had a discussion of the treatment which was to begin on Friday. I asked Buddy about limitations on Sandy's activities, mentioning that we had played tennis that afternoon. All four doctors were astonished and Buddy exclaimed curtly, "Sidney, she only has 10 grams of hemoglobin. I don't see how she ever got on the tennis court. No more tennis." But in time all of them came to recognize the spirit that Sandy had and to treat her in keeping with that spirit rather than merely as a "leukemia." It was decided to meet with Sandy on Friday afternoon to discuss the findings and plan for the treatment of her "anemia." Transfusions and medication had to begin immediately.

Friday morning began cold and gray, with mist and some rain blurring the windows. Sandy put Russell in his bassinet and changed his diapers. She gave him a tickle on his stomach and then asked me to carry him downstairs for breakfast. Propping him in her arms at the kitchen table she spooned little bits of Pablum from a jar on the marble table-top into his mouth and talked about the day before us and whether we should go to the Opera Society party that night. She worked in public relations for the Opera Society and her committee was planning a great newspaper spread for the next production. She had to be fitted for a dress and have pictures taken for the following Sunday's newspapers.

"I'll need the little red car this morning to go down and have my picture taken for some Opera Society publicity. I can meet you down at Buddy's after lunch," Sandy said. "Why does he want to see us both anyway?"

"He said he wanted to explain it to both of us so we would both know the plan and be able to go ahead with it," I told her.

"What is the plan? I don't see why there is all this planning. I'll just have to take some iron pills or something for a while."

We'd finished our espresso. Sandy gave me a warm kiss, straightened my tie, and said, "You look so handsome today, darling." When I left she held Russell in her arms and waved his little hand at mine through the window.

I went to Children's Hospital, then to Catholic University to give a lecture on the psychology of adolescence. This was a two-hour lecture to a group of one hundred social work students. As I spoke of the need for independence and rebellion in adolescence, the adolescent's hunger for sensation and experience, I caught myself gazing out the window and losing track of my notes occasionally. My eyes focused momentarily on the great new Cathedral of the Immaculate Conception with its sparkling blue-and-yellow mosaic dome but then quickly returned to rebellion and independence. After the lecture I hurried over to the basilica and, kneeling in its vast emptiness, reflected about what to do. I was searching everywhere for direction at that time, though direction was elusive. Then, hurrying home, which, I suppose, was the direction, I had lunch with Sandy, kissed Russell, and drove to the doctors' offices.

We all sat in Buddy's office, little birds on a branch, and the conference began. Buddy introduced Dr. Ed Adelson, Dr. Jack Rheingold and Dr. Arnold Lear to Sandy. They all were extremely competent hematologists or blood specialists who, to our good fortune, shared the same suite of offices with Dr. Gusack. Sandy was a bit bewildered by the seriousness of the discussion, my nodding in agreement, and Buddy's saying, "All of us will be here any time, Sandy dear. But Arnold Lear will be the one you'll see regularly because he knows most about treating this kind of anemia."

"What kind of anemia is it?" Sandy asked.

Ed Adelson began to speak, but Buddy interrupted. "Well, it's just because you don't have enough red blood cells and we need to build up your blood."

"Was it because of the baby?"

"Sandy, we don't know what it was caused by. We do know we have to treat it right away and treat it vigorously. We'll give you some medicine to take today and then do a transfusion tomorrow morning."

"How do I take the medicine?"

"They're just pills. Sidney can get them at Morgan's. I'll call right away." And, characteristically, in the middle of our discussion, Buddy lifted the phone and called Morgan's Pharmacy to tell them what he wanted. Thus began the inclusion of one of the few small, intimate drugstores left in Washington in the design. The pharmacist at Morgan's knew Sandy and Russell by name and always gave Niccolo a malt tablet on Sunday morning when we walked there to pick up the *New York Times*. Most of the orders he filled were for lipstick, Roger & Gallet soap and all the other things women need. Now he heard the prescription for Prednisone, 6-mercaptopurine and methotrexate. Prednisone sometimes is given for asthma or minor skin difficulties, but methotrexate and 6-mercaptopurine are desperate medications, used only against the most deadly blood cancers. The pharmacist never discussed the medications with Sandy and she never asked. I tried to pick up the refill prescriptions myself, but there were a number of times when Sandy blithely sailed into Morgan's and got the paper bags filled with medicines, like a go-between in a spy thriller, not knowing what was in the envelopes.

Sandy became restive at being a part of all the head nodding and discussions of blood cells and blood production. Finally, she said, "You know, I'm feeling a lot better already." She held my hand tightly, looked around, and said, "Maybe I could put off taking the medicine for a while to see whether my body's defenses can get themselves better on their own."

"That's a possibility," Jack Rheingold quickly replied, "but we can't take the chance involved in not treating you."

We then ended the joint interview and Sandy went off to talk with Arnold Lear about an appointment to return the next morning for a transfusion. She left the office that afternoon as a patient with a serious illness committed to a perilous course.

She began that evening shoveling three tablets of one medicine, four of another down her throat, murmuring ruefully, "It must be one large anemia, for me to have to take all this." We sat quietly at dinner, feebly joking about whether the medicine had changed her already, and went to bed early in preparation for the transfusion Saturday.

It took about three hours for the transfusion of two pints of blood to be completed the next morning. During the procedure, I wandered down to St. John's Episcopal Church, which we attended on Sundays, and sat there for a while. But I realized that I've always believed religion is for the healthy, to remind strong people to do good works for others, not to heal the lame and the sick. It was a meandering, thoughtless time.

On Sunday, we drove to Towson, Maryland, past lovely autumn colors in the Maryland hunt country to visit with a psychiatrist friend. When we greeted each other, he asked Sandy how she was.

"Well, I have an anemia and just had a transfusion yesterday," she answered straightforwardly.

He replied, "I'm so sorry to hear that. I went to

see a colleague while he was getting a transfusion
on Thursday. He died yesterday and the funeral is
Monday. The poor devil had leukemia and he died
in two weeks."

I boggled at this and tried to turn the conversation to other things, but he asked what kind of anemia Sandy had. She told him it was due to not having enough red blood cells and that her body was
not making enough blood.

It is remarkable that, when we are not thinking
directly about a subject, we accept the most artless
explanations of complicated problems. He, truly,
didn't take in what he would have understood in a
moment if he had been thinking medically and, instead, turned to show us his house and the lovely
view down the long group of knolls to a stand of
oak trees.

On Monday photographers posed Sandy in a
friend's house for more Opera Society publicity.
She liked the dress she was given to wear and was
pleased that she looked so slim. I kidded her at dinner about being in another man's house, but then
glumness set in. We had done all the proper things,
got started on the medicine, experienced all the
drama. Now we were to wait and improvise,
though I had two more people yet to appeal to.

Chapter 6

 I continued to look for a way we could get some magical help in this fearful time, for my training as a doctor had been too effective for there to be any remnant of hope that the disease could be cured or the diagnosis shown to be a ludicrous mistake. Sandy's physicians were simply too capable to have made such a mistake. Good doctors rarely make diagnostic errors, which is unfortunate, for patients love to dream of fooling their physicians. Well-trained physicians may give too little medicine on occasion, forget to take a bandage off, or neglect to examine a patient's eyes, but they never miss leukemia. All of my medical life I had witnessed the opposite — the most accurate and devastating diagnoses and predictions of the outcome of disease.

So I looked elsewhere, further into the realm of the spirit. The people I thought of were the minister of our church and the man who had been my psychoanalyst. During psychiatric training many doctors are psychoanalyzed, some to learn how to be psychoanalysts themselves, some because of personal problems, and some for both reasons. I had gone through this process several years before and had profited a good deal from it. It was quite natural for me to think of going back to talk with my psychoanalyst. When I called him he made a particular effort to change his schedule and see me quickly. Hoping there might be some answer, somewhere, I began to tell him my now familiar story.

"Sandy has acute granulocytic leukemia. I just wondered if there is anything I can do about it," I said.

He began to question me. "What do the cells look like? How sure are they about the diagnosis? Has she lost much blood?"

I answered the questions, but my replies became increasingly automatic.

Then he asked what everyone asks about leukemia patients.

"Isn't it possible that she has a number of years to live?"

I tried to tell him I hoped so, that there was a chance, but my voice wandered off. I was thinking that any prediction of a finite end, no matter how benevolent, was no comfort. When such a prediction is made, the clock of death starts ticking more clearly than before. I didn't want to hear that clock at all, that is, not until death itself came. That kind of ticking makes life a time bomb instead of a celebration; it puts dread into every moment. So I changed the subject.

"I really came to talk with you to see if I can figure out any way to be strong and helpful to Sandy during the time that's left," I said. After a few more desultory interchanges, what I later began to call "the" question came, one that recurred in people's thoughts and inquiries until the end — "Does she know?"

Patiently I tried to explain Buddy's view and mine, that we had to wait for a definitive diagnosis and the proper moment. But I spared him my real reaction, that this question was already becoming an impertinence to my mind, merely an aspect of morbid curiosity.

But, liking him very much and appreciative of his concern and all that he had done for me, I turned our conversation to proper psychological observations.

"On the first night this happened," I reported, "after she fell asleep, she called out in her sleep, 'How is Russell? I think I hear him. Take care of Russell.' "

"So she does know," he said, as if that made any difference. Then he added, "Do you have a good person to take care of Russell? How are you taking it?" Question after question came.

Though I appreciated immensely his courtesy and kindness, I could see that he was rooted in a reality different from mine. He just didn't have the willingness or ability to soar, to say anything remarkable. Such an ability is beyond most of us, although some people do have it. It is a combination of words and tone, of searching optimism and greathearted charm. It is Les Glenn's saying "For her it should be forty years from now," and then speaking in his affirmative voice about his belief in faith. It is Marshal Lyautey saying that if he knew a certain seedling would not mature for a hundred years, it must be planted immediately.

What I needed to hear again and again was the literal absurdity of Sandy's illness, not, at that time, questions about reality. And so I thanked him and began to leave. He called after me, "I'll be glad to see you at any time. If there is anything I can do . . ."

I then appealed to the last person on my list, the rector of our church in Washington. To say that he was decent and kind is to say the obvious, but, again, I hoped for more. By the time I walked into his study on the second floor of the church building, I had become a bit more sophisticated in the tactics of asking for the impossible.

I had learned that you ask, not for what you really want, but for tokens — the names of books, the experiences of others, a way of organizing time, the rituals one must go through. Fortunately, I passed through this phase quickly, but I did have to experience it before I could return to a world of simplicity and fairy tales.

We settled down in easy chairs in the rector's study, chaffing each other about how difficult it was for us to get together about other matters that concerned us. He spoke about how important psychiatry was to his work, and we reminisced about Russell's christening before I began my story.

"Sandy has a serious illness, leukemia. Her doctors don't know how long she will live, and I've been trying to think of some way to figure out the time we have left." There was silence, so I added, "I wondered about going to Florida or Europe, or something."

He replied, "No, I wouldn't go to Florida or Europe, at least not for a long trip."

We engaged in several more conventional interchanges, followed by the predictable question, "Do you have someone to care for the baby?"

I decided it was time to ask about books. He suggested John Baillie's *A Diary of Readings*, as had Les Glenn, and as everyone else would in answer to my inquiry. I said I would get the book, but it seemed very curious then, as it does now, that there is such a small shelf of works that can be recommended to people in despair. He offered to come to the house to visit Sandy and said other thoughtful things as I took my leave. But he spoke of organization, when I needed poetry.

Now my rounds were over. There was no place else to appeal. Unlike an appellant in the legal system, I couldn't seek redress from a higher court. But, it was a fair batting average, one hit and two misses. And how blessed Sandy and I were that we, at least, had people to appeal to.

It was fortunate that I was a psychiatrist and could call on the warm concern of another psychiatrist, and a blessing that the church as an institution was there to try to fathom the depths of inevitability. Though both institutions, religion and psychiatry, did not speak to me at those moments, perhaps they do to others in similar moments, and perhaps they will speak more clearly and easily to all in the future.

What does one hope for at such times? My great hope was for transformation, magic, that Sandy's illness would vanish and she would become healthy again. We have lived too long with Cinderella and Snow White and the Ugly Duckling to hope for less. Somehow, when lost inside a black, dark cavern, we hope for an ascension, a miracle.

Actually, I was looking for that little bit more, that willingness to be awed, that ability to smile and speak of faith, the directness that cries "Horseshit!" at conventional answers, an interest in arguing or crying or getting inside the head of another person.

Perhaps the time will come when institutions can respond and help. In the meantime we all depend upon God's spies on this earth, those originals who, in a time of maximal need, offer simply everything — the Les Glenns, the Buddy Gusacks, and a few others.

Chapter 7

 Five days after the diagnosis was made Sandy was still alive. Transfusions and a bone marrow aspiration had been completed and she swallowed three different varieties of pills every six hours. I spoke with Buddy only once a day and heard the white count and red-blood-cell count readings — not better, but, far more important, not worse. A routine, however shaky and potentially macabre, settled over our lives, and we could think of Russell and his nurse Gloria and our ordinary interests a bit.

Despite the slight easing from the initial shock and horror and disbelief, the unspeakable idea of death and the phrase "fatal illness" pervaded my mind, like the constant A that Robert Schumann heard sounding in his ear.

What do you think and do? Often, I froze into a vacant stare for long moments when alone, and then roused myself to try to invent some kind of plan that would keep us afloat. Hectic thoughts of travel came first. If we could only go back to Arcetri, that tiny village hung high above Florence beyond San Miniato, where Sandy appeared one morning, never to leave again. In my daydreams I saw us walking down under the gray rainy sky past the little espresso shop, where coffee was served in tiny glasses and tasted as good as it did at Bruzzichelli in the Piazza del Duomo in the center of Florence. Then to the fruit man, who always had a bright *"Buon giorno"* and happy words about the peaches and oranges that stood in pyramids outside his store. The walls of the long row of four stores, including our favorite restaurant, Omero, were still covered with aging, cracking signs from the time of Mussolini, proclaiming: *Fascisti, uniti, pace,* and other inanities.

Even though it was pleasant to consider a trip to Italy, retreating there would have solved no problems but only have offered us a way to climb into a coffin and pull the lid down on us. Boca Grande, Florida, with its warm sun and long beaches covered with conch shells and periwinkles also called to me. But that would take up only a few weeks

and we would become bored. All the other possibilities — Jamaica, the Virgin Islands, Maine,
crazy possibilities such as Jesselton, in North Bor-
neo, or the Ivory Coast, all brought back memories
of delight or interesting Peace Corps work, but
offered no reality to us. And, for me, even at this
moment, reflecting back on that now distant time,
I realize that the only place I wanted ever to be
was close to Sandy and holding her hand or tracing
a soft pattern on the back of her wrist.

Practical issues intruded on this daydreaming,
too. I was treating patients and couldn't very well
stop work with them. They needed me and, in a
very definite way, I needed them, for I found that
concentration on the problems of patients helped
me to forget my own, at least temporarily. The
thought of moving from Washington just did not fit
in with my professional responsibilities.

The cost of travel or, for that matter, the cost of
any of the extra burdens of Sandy's illness never
became serious considerations in our decisions.
From the beginning of our marriage Sandy and I
gave each other the gift of not talking or worrying
about money. We were prudent in most things,
though we seldom held back on extravagances
such as trips to New York, books, flowers or presents. When leukemia became the principal focus

of life, even fleeting preoccupations with money seemed irrelevant. We lived in the moment in all ways and the major factor in the decision to remain where we were was not financial but Sandy's need to stay close to pipettes, blood-counting apparatus and doctors who knew her medical condition intimately. If we moved away from Washington a medical misstep might occur, and even a slight misstep could be fatal.

But her life was ending nonetheless, and I searched my mind endlessly for a thought or plan that might lighten the weight of such an awful finality.

Plans appeared in my mind and then vanished as ordinary life continued for us. Often I sat in the kitchen and watched, mesmerized, as Sandy fed Russell his Pablum. She would laugh and coo with him as she turned his wide silver spoon upward in his mouth to steer the last few morsels of the gruelly stuff against his upper lip so it would remain inside his mouth and not become streaked across his cheeks. And then she would arrange flowers on the marble kitchen table before she placed them around the living room. Suddenly a thought would leap into my mind of lying quietly on a beach on the island of Kos in Greece, looking over toward Bodrum and the great, red Turkish mountains that loomed through the warm, misty dawn from the east. Sandy and I should be there, I mused, but then I would remember that I had to see a patient at my office at Children's Hospital and, at the same time, arrange transportation for Sandy to Buddy's office.

A further demand of reality was that of keeping Sandy's family in Boston informed of her disease. Her brothers, Harry and Jimmy, and their wives, and her sister Ellen and Ellen's husband, were extremely close and loving, so I phoned Jimmy shortly after the definite diagnosis was made and spoke with him frequently during the first weeks. Then I wrote him the following letter to summarize where we were:

November 14, 1966

Dear Jimmy,

This has been a time of the most dreadful news. I have been so caught up in it that there hasn't been a chance to write you. But you might want to hear what has happened on paper in preparation for the moment when it will be best to tell your mother and father. Naturally, share this with Harry and Lisa at any time, also with Ellen and Tom. I haven't written them or called because it is so painful to be reminded of what is happening over and over again. It was a great support to me to be able to talk with you over the last several weeks. Without your ear to share this with, I don't know if I could have kept my end up here.

At the time of Russell's christening, Sandy had a cold and a low-grade fever. On Wednesday, October 26th, she went in to see her doctor for a checkup and to discover why the fever had persisted. Frankly, I expected nothing to be uncovered; neither did Dr. Gusack. He saw her, found nothing, and sent her home. However, he took a blood test and that afternoon his lab technician told him there were leukemia cells in Sandy's blood. He checked it himself, then called in some colleagues. He shares his office with Drs. Rheingold, Lear and Adelson, some of the finest hematologists in Washington. All of them have been trained by Dr. Dameshek, the world's authority on blood diseases, particularly leukemia. They looked at the slides and there was no doubt about the diagnosis.

They brought Sandy back the next day for an aspiration of blood from her bone marrow. This test totally corroborated their findings. She has what is called Acute Granulocytic Leukemia. In this disease the white blood cells have gone haywire for no known reason. They take over and prevent red blood cells from forming. It is the most deadly kind of leukemia.

She was immediately started on intensive treatment to try to stop the growth of the abnormal white cells. Fortunately, the treatment is not painful, consisting of taking many pills by mouth. Sandy has been doing that for more than two weeks now.

They sent the slides to Dr. Dameshek, who has moved from Boston to New York, to Dr. Cravens at Johns Hopkins, and to Colonel Crosby, who is now in Boston. The diagnosis was confirmed by them and the treatment totally agreed upon.

71

Sandy has felt a bit weak and has looked pale. But she continues to take care of Russell, to teach one day a week, and to visit with friends. For example, we went to Baltimore yesterday and had a very happy visit with Mrs. Crimmins. We go to the movies, occasionally go out to dinner, and have had a most happy time together. She is in fine spirits and very courageous.

There has been some slight good news. There are now fewer "blast" cells, the immature abnormal white cells, in her blood. However, because she developed increasing anemia, she went in to the doctor today and was given two units of packed red blood cells by transfusion this afternoon. To emphasize how strange the whole thing is, we had a fine dinner and evening tonight and she is going down to the Opera Society to do some work tomorrow.

I hate to share this with you, but it is so awful that, except for a miracle, a year or two are considered long survival times. Fortunately, with the drugs being used, she may feel absolutely perfect in two or three weeks and remain in excellent health for months.

That is why I haven't told her what she has, nor have her doctors. They feel very strongly that it only adds to the burden of illness when she is feeling pretty well. Also, when it first happened, I realized in talking with her that she wanted hope, not doom. I would have wanted the same, and I still do. I don't feel at all that this is deception but rather a decent humanity. When she really wants to know, her doctors will tell her. I might add that they are very warm and fine people as well as excellent physicians. She trusts them and feels very comfortable in going down to their offices.

I will keep you informed. We hope to come to Boston
for Christmas.

All my love to Buffy, Beth, and you,
Sidney

Chapter 8

 Sandy's life revolved around the medicine she swallowed every few hours, the tip of a transfusion needle and little boxes that examined her blood and produced numbers that determined whether she had enough red blood cells to allow her to breathe comfortably.

Our life was circumscribed by Ray, who drew Sandy's blood so deftly, Miss Atkinson, the receptionist who made us feel welcome with a "How nice to see you today," and Mrs. Anderson, always ready with a warm "Hi there, Mrs. Werkman. Dr. Gusack will see you just as soon as he gets off the phone." As soon as the danger of an immediate death passed, Sandy returned to teaching at the Potomac School, a country day school in Virginia. She came home at night to tell of unruly students, mostly boys, projectors that didn't work in her French class geared to a new teaching method, and the teacher gossip of a lively faculty. We resumed our tempo of Thursday dinner parties at our house, morning music making with piano and flute, and delight in our son Russell, who was changing from being a little pug-nosed baby into a mature, subtle half-year-old with yellow, almost white, eyebrows and beginning freckles.

Sandy's native good humor and decisiveness helped her enormously during her illness. Her mother told me, "During summer vacation time when Sandy was a youngster, she was always the first one up and dressed for morning tennis. She always got the car because she knew what she wanted to do the entire day when the other children were still groggy from sleep." The pattern continued throughout her adult life. Her Bryn Mawr college yearbook sketch attests to that. Some anonymous biographer wrote this of her in the 1960 yearbook:

Goooood morning! Windows bang, covers are thrown back. Before we're out of bed, Sandy has washed, dressed, breakfasted, made her bed, and is studying. Wrinkling her nose, she belies her angelic appearance with an emphatic " °°°°," as she leaves medieval history for fifteen laps in the pool. Then a quick change

75

from chlorine to "Miss Dior," and Sandy's off for another football weekend.

And, if I reach further back, to the cruder prose of a boarding school yearbook, the 1956 *Ragged Robin* of the Garrison Forest School in Maryland, the same theme comes through:

Even on the coldest days found wearing only her blazer and SPS [St. Paul's School] scarf over her uniform. Giving expert advice about knitting. Always thinking up new things to worry about. Complete unsophistication. In a frenzy over yearbook pictures. Fresh as a daisy look. Pompom on her hat in constant motion. Hair that naturally does what it's supposed to. Using three straws at milk and crackers. Authentic French accent. Nightly use of dental floss. Earnest, dependable and cheerful. Famous for: Her walk.

During her illness Sandy took on many opportunities to use her cheerful energy, but she also made her opportunities. Because both of us loved opera — my father sang "Là ci darem la mano" in a good baritone voice every day of my life, following that with "Che gelida manina," oblivious to the need to change from his natural baritone to a slightly falsetto tenor — Sandy was delighted to be a vice-president of the Washington Opera Society. In that post she presided at women's teas in embassies, licked stamps for mailings in the Society's offices, was privy to the politics of opera, which made up a fair amount of our dinner conversation, and, almost as an afterthought, attended openings and parties for the openings.

As we sat in our living room before dinner one evening with Russell between us on a sofa, Sandy said, tentatively, "Darling, Mrs. Williams called up today and asked if I would be a vice-president of the Kennedy Center. She wants Linda Coles and me to be the young ones, so we can get some other people our age working for the center." She spoke of arranging for tours of the site just then taking shape into the vast complex it would become, and of planning benefits so that children could be admitted free to concerts and opera when the whole center opened. "Do you think I should try it?" she asked.

For the first time I had to begin to weigh probabilities and realities in tangible compartments of days, and months, and balance them against the potent harm they might do to her health. I was no longer thinking only of when Sandy would die; a subtle change of focus and planning had taken place.

"Can she get through to Christmas? Maybe the Kennedy Center work will be interesting for her," I thought. And I never questioned whether activity might hurt her, for those lethal corpuscles were not going to go away and death would be better if it came quickly and without pain, rather than after a long, losing struggle with increasing discomfort and loss of strength.

So I replied, "Of course you should do it." Sandy was pleased, and reminded me, "I think your father would be happy about my doing it too, because he loves opera so much."

Her appointment book shows how she interspersed doctors and transfusions casually between cocktail parties and Opera Society meetings without missing many heartbeats of life. The book contains one more example of her thoughtfulness. She arranged for Gloria and Elena, a friend of Gloria's, to go to the opera together.

I continued my career, which centered on the psychiatry department at Children's Hospital in Washington. Every day I taught students and residents in psychiatry, gave seminars, and treated patients. But almost always, as I participated in a State Department conference on Youth in Developing Countries or gave lectures, there was the mind-stopping thought of the cells I had seen under a microscope on October 26th.

If I forgot for a while or was lulled into delighted complacency by the now normal warmth of

Sandy's arm next to mine in bed, the awful knowledge returned abruptly every time we journeyed
down to Buddy Gusack's office for another hematocrit determination or a transfusion, and every
time he made one of his regular Tuesday late-after-
noon visits to our house on his way home with his
nurse, Mrs. Anderson, to see us and have tea and
cookies.

At the door as I was saying good-bye, or, at
times, at his office while I waited for the last dripping of blood into Sandy's arm during a transfusion, Buddy and I would have a hurried word
together, a confrontation with each other's knowledge, and those moments were always ones of
stunned blankness on my part and poignant omis-
sions on his. Though we both shared a kind of Russian fatalism, he always outmaneuvered me, even
when I wanted to feel most heartbroken. He repeated himself on the same subject a number of
times, as busy people do, when I looked most hap-
less.

"Cousin," he would remind me with a smile and
matter-of-fact animation, "some people have lived
for ten years with acute granulocytic. Maybe
Sandy will. She's doing well now."

"But not many," I would shoot back.

His voice would falter then, but he would recover and quickly ask about our plans for Thanksgiving or tell me about a patient we both knew, and I would forget the awful finality as he slipped out the door with a pat on my shoulder.

Who knows how our lives would have formed over the years? Certainly we would continue to pack up our swimsuits and tennis rackets each March and go to Jamaica or Florida for several weeks to shake off the long winter and get in shape for spring tennis; then a month on Cape Cod in the summer, occasional years in Europe. I hoped always to do more writing, for I liked the process and the occasional delight of seeing words strung together. Sandy enjoyed teaching and worked hard at developing new materials to interest her students of French. She practiced the piano and tried to find ways to make her activities on volunteer committees helpful to poor and sick children. We shared a wish to help develop a medical school in Iran or Pakistan and, in her insistent, quiet way, she was the main force behind this wish, for she felt a kind of obligation to do original things in life. But all that was now in the past, and we had to invent new, more immediate possibilities to keep ourselves afloat.

Chapter 9

 I felt we couldn't survive the daily closeness of Washington unless we could find some safety valves, for there were too many jarring, incompatible experiences mixed together in the attempt to keep up a semblance of a usual life. Most of those experiences centered on blood counts and transfusions. Sandy's hemoglobin level veered crazily from 12 grams to 4 grams in several days. The Friday morning after Thanksgiving it bottomed at 4 grams, and another transfusion was ordered immediately. Small matters in comparison to death, but, after a delightful Thanksgiving-night supper for "foreigners" (English, French, and Italian) with a flawlessly accented reading by one guest of Art Buchwald's classic dissertation on Thanksgiving for

the French, the ominously low hemoglobin set off a
battle-station bell, meaning cancellation of Gloria's
day off so she could take care of Russell, changing
patient appointments at the hospital in the afternoon for me, and compressing a two-hour lecture
at Catholic University into one, so I could be near
Sandy. The possibility of a transfusion reaction
gripped me, and always, always, the possibility
that the blood would not help hovered in my
thoughts.

Like most of the grisly ghosts of the night, my
fears were dissipated when the last few drops of
blood plop-plopped, the needle was slipped out of
Sandy's elbow vein, and a cotton puff, followed by
a round Band-Aid, was applied. On Sandy's part
the whole operation was accepted with patience,
and she wondered aloud about which dress to wear
to the opening of the opera that evening.

By midafternoon Sandy was free of all the transfusion tubing and she walked out of Buddy Gusack's office on my arm. As we drove home, she
asked, "Darling, would you be an angel and stop at
the shoemaker's and ask if they can dye a pair of
shoes the color of my dress for tonight? And I have
to tell Annie that we are coming to the party for
Rodiga and Carlos before we go to dinner."

We did get the shoes, go to cocktails, dinner, a pleasant performance of *Werther,* and even stopped in for a moment at the Austrian Embassy reception afterward.

Everything seemed to be going well and happily, but the disease was progressing, for Sandy had just received a transfusion on Tuesday.

On the morning after the opera, we began the activity that sustained us more than anything else during the months of Sandy's illness. Several weeks before, I paid a call on Mrs. Poe Burling, "Ella," a longtime friend. In the fashion afforded only by a city such as Washington, organized around dinner parties where extra men and women are needed, Ella and I were seated next to each other many times. We danced together at Sulgrave Club parties and saw each other at Sunday lunches in the country. On Sandy's family's side, Ella was a friend, hostess and contemporary of Mr. and Mrs. Colt, with ties between them stretching back to World War II, Harvard and, so far as I knew, infinity.

So it was no great leap to visit her and ask her advice and a potential favor. My only concern was about whether to tell her the extent of Sandy's illness. As we sat in a corner of her living room, had coffee, and chatted about how Russell was thriving, Ella may have thought I was going to speak about family difficulties or a new intrigue in the Opera Society. After a brief answer to her "Sidney, how is that dear little baby of yours?" I launched directly into my concern.

"Sandy is very sick. She has a very serious anemia."

"But she will recover . . ." Ella answered, uncertainly. "I know you can get her to the finest doctors." And, after a pause, "What can I help you with?"

"I'd like to find a place away from Washington I can take Sandy off to on weekends," I said. "I've looked into West Virginia property and little houses in Virginia, but right now we just don't have the energy to buy a place and then have to get it fixed as we want it. I wondered if you knew of any houses on the Eastern Shore we might rent, or even if your little guesthouse on the Eastern Shore might be available for us to rent this winter."

"Oh, Sidney, someone has the guesthouse, but you must have the big house. I'm going to be away most of the winter and my handyman will take good care of you." A few more arrangements, "thank you's" and meshing of times, and we had a house in the country.

On the last Saturday morning of November, surprisingly warm for that time of year, we packed extra diapers for Russell, old sweaters, some food, Gloria's television set, and we set off for the Eastern Shore of Maryland. We drove fast to get there at midmorning, across the Chesapeake Bay Bridge arching to the sky, then to the right toward St. Michaels, Maryland, and to Claiborne. St. Michaels has a main street, but Claiborne consists solely of a single store — gasoline station, general store, post office and town hall all in one — and several houses. I knew we had found what we needed, even before we sighted the twin brick pillars of Ella's house. Beyond the pillars the front lawn, studded sparsely with enormous, gracious oaks, stretched lazily to the Chesapeake Bay. The house itself was a blessing from the moment we entered its dark hall and explored the high-ceilinged, octagonal living room and vast, cold kitchen. We unpacked hurriedly, put on bathing suits, and had lunch beside the swimming pool in the good autumn warmth of a direct sun in a cloudless sky. While Gloria and I played with Russell on the front lawn, Sandy fell into a serene sleep beside the pool. Later we moved inside because it turned cold quickly at midafternoon, and we listened to the opera on an old, bulky all-wave Zenith portable radio that stuttered over New York but brought in Greece and Afghanistan adequately, while Russell crawled along the red-carpeted floor in a jumble of checkers, backgammon counters and poker chips.

Before the weekend was finished we walked across long, flat cornfields to the Bay, explored fishing boats, stopped along the beach and sent stones splashing into the water, and sat blissfully before the warming fires. I treasure a particular picture of Sandy from that first weekend, a photograph of her bounding along, wearing a blue and gray Loden coat she bought on a trip to Aspen, Colorado, the previous autumn, hands clasped in the small of her back, head up, and hair brushed awry by a slight wind.

The delicious quietness of dinner on trays, happily alone with our small family — Russell worming about on the floor, Niccolo sniffing every corner, and Gloria happily bringing in rice and sharing our wine — formed moments we enjoyed many times and always with gratefulness. Though we slept in a room with twin beds, I moved over in the early morning to Sandy's bed with its somewhat bowed mattress, and we fell together perfectly and quietly, nuzzling each other awake. Those moments of utter peace, perfection, the moments beyond tragedy, the great moments when all time, all thought were obliterated, gave us the strength to withstand most of the storms that lay ahead.

Chapter 10

 Sandy was just four days free of transfusions when we drove back to Washington. After her first appointment with Dr. Lear on Monday, he called me to say her blood picture was not going well. A lot of blast cells had returned to her peripheral blood and she was quite anemic; her hemoglobin level had dropped precipitously to 6 grams. Another transfusion was necessary at midweek and, more disheartening to Sandy, the dosage of drugs, particularly methotrexate and 6-mercaptopurine, was increased.

"What do the blasts mean?" I asked, half knowing the answer.

Arnold replied, "We can't be sure, but probably, the remission is over."

"Will there be another one?" I asked.

"There could be, but she had such a good response to the methotrexate and 6-mercaptopurine the first time, we'll have to see and maybe change her drugs. Would you like to talk to Buddy about it?"

After talking with Arnold and then Buddy and Ed Adelson, I confirmed what I knew anyway from reading textbooks on blood diseases at the Children's Hospital library. Those drugs, available only in the last ten years, were one-time winners. In the past anyone with Sandy's variety of leukemia, acute granulocytic leukemia, could expect to die within days or a few months of diagnosis. With the use of cortisone-like drugs, Prednisone being one of them, survival time often was increased by a number of months. But Prednisone does not produce a total reversal of the disease process. That is, it never rids the blood of the overflow of young or immature white blood cells, the ones that give the disease its name — leukemia, or "white blood." Instead, the drug helps the patient feel more comfortable and has only a slight direct effect on the blood elements themselves.

When methotrexate and 6-mercaptopurine were discovered, the treatment of leukemia took a new turn. These drugs produce, in favorable cases, one clean, often complete, reversal, but they seldom work a second time. Also, they are powerful poisons and have the potential for destroying all the elements of the blood and causing the immediate death of a patient. So, the hematologist has to gamble on what is best in each case. Should he give a patient Prednisone and hope she will live a long time, that is, many months, but have a slow, regular decline, or should he try the new drugs and run the risk of killing his patient while playing for the stakes of a return to good health for a miraculous period of time?

Sandy's doctors chose to gamble and I agreed totally with their plan. They had won, for Sandy did get her strength and delight in life back for more than a month. She gained some weight again and felt optimistic about the future. But that particular wager was now paid off and the dreaded blast cells were floating around in her body again. This time the chance of destroying them with drugs was much slimmer.

This realization made the prospect of Christmas and any kind of future thought and planning less appealing, and it turned my mind to final thoughts and some kind of plan that would soften the death I was expecting in the next month or so.

Since we had given up the idea of any exotic travels, our choices seemed limited to staying in

Washington throughout Christmas or making a dash for Boston. Neither alternative was attractive, for I saw Boston as the last resort, the place we would try to get to when nothing else was left, and Washington, during a period of decline, would be a torturing experience.

Fortunately, Sandy and I flew to New York just before Christmas every year so I could attend the meeting of the American Psychoanalytic Association, and we both could visit friends, see plays, and buy Christmas presents. I chose this pleasant plan now as a way to take our minds from the inexorable movement of the disease. I thought of the trip as a special one, for I didn't believe Sandy would ever be able to have another spree. Though many of the adjustments she made to illness were tiny ones, they all added up to a great change in her life. She took a long time to dress in the morning and wasn't able to push Russell in his baby carriage or carry packages; she needed long naps every afternoon and couldn't walk more than a few steps without feeling extremely tired. I decided to go all out on the trip. We would rent a limousine, buy glittering presents, and in one weekend fulfill wishes usually spread out over a lifetime. Then we could return to Washington in good spirits to look straight at the *real* prospect of our lives.

We flew up to LaGuardia Airport from Washington on a gray, drizzly morning and were met by a car and chauffeur I had arranged as a great surprise. Instead of our waiting for bags and a porter and a cab, everything was taken care of in a moment and we sped off over the Triborough Bridge into the clogged, sleek, dirty, brilliant, separate world of Manhattan. First, we went to Bergdorf's to buy some presents for nieces. During the morning and early afternoon the car stopped at Brooks Brothers, Abercrombie's and Schwarz's for toys.

But the great treat was a visit to Bendel's fur shop after our quick tour of Bergdorf's. The car, waiting at the Fifth Avenue curb, made a circle to get on Fifty-seventh Street and deposited us at Bendel's, where we were ushered into a quiet room high in the store with a window looking out on Fifty-seventh Street. Sandy was tired and hungry, so the manager quickly arranged to have orange juice, coffee and croissants brought. He introduced us to a pretty woman with black hair and a warm smile, who looked like my mother. "Mrs. Railes will take excellent care of you," he said and then disappeared.

Mrs. Railes took over. "Everyone calls me Mary," she said immediately. Her warm statement reminded me of the first line of the lovely opening soprano aria in *La Bohème*, Mi chiamano Mimì — They call me Mimi — and I knew we were going to have a good time.

Mary brought out a number of fur coats, had models demonstrate them, and then wore them herself. Sandy tried on several of them, before both of us became entranced with a particularly lovely high-collared black muskrat coat. We decided on it instantly.

Sandy sank into a deep silk sofa, somewhat tired, but flushed with delight over her first fur coat. The fitter made some tentative pinnings for small alterations that needed to be done. He then asked what kind of lining she wanted — white, gray, black, silver, gold? A gold lining with an *A* faintly woven into it was chosen.

Since we were going to the opera that night, Sandy wanted very much to wear the coat.

Miss Mary was taken aback. "We can't get it ready for you tonight, even next week will be difficult. But, I can help you out. I'll have the lining pinned in myself, just so you can wear it to the opera tonight, but you must bring it back to me in the morning, so we can put the lining in properly and make all the changes you need. I'll have it mailed to Washington next week, unless you would prefer to come back to New York for another fitting."

We were delighted with the plan to have the coat sent to Washington and arranged to have our driver return in the afternoon to pick it up for use that evening.

The limousine threaded its way through the tiny streets of the Village and deposited us, our arms filled with luggage and colorfully wrapped Christmas packages, at the house of Sandy's aunt and uncle. After we had a long nap and happy dinner, Uncle Chis, knowing of Sandy's illness, arranged for another limousine to take us to the Metropolitan Opera. In his irrepressible way, he looked at his niece's new fur coat, jutted his chin high in the air, laughed his hearty laugh, and said, "That's just a *dandy* coat." We rollicked off to the opera, through rain-cleaned streets, and swept into the new opera house for a performance of *Aïda* with Richard Tucker and Leontyne Price. Champagne between acts strengthened us for the dying falls of the Tomb Scene at the end with its love duet between Radames and Aïda, dying in each other's arms.

Uncle Chis was the first one to speak. "That was a perfectly *marvelous* production." And then the magic of the opera was continued into the real magic of the night still to come. We got back to Uncle Chis's house on MacDougal Street in a most exhilarated state, had a brandy together, and went off to our bed. Sandy and I slept in a bedroom fronting on MacDougal Street and were treated, as always, to the night noises of that raucous place. She had put on her nightgown, brushed her hair just as if she were still in boarding school, and prepared for bed. We fell into bed close to each other and made love.

Sandy no longer took contraceptive pills because they masked the effect of all the other hormonal medication she was taking. In fact, back in September the first hint of her illness had been an irregularity in her menstrual periods and a problem in being able to use contraceptive pills effectively. As a result she had never returned to the regular use of pills after Russell was born.

We knew there was some concern about pregnancy, but who could consider such a possibility when death was a more real one? According to the malignant schedule of her disease, to last long enough to buy a fur coat and go to the opera in New York at Christmas was a gift, and I thought of the New Year as an impossibly long time away.

Now, when bliss overcame us and we lay tranquilly listening to the dampened clamor outside before we fell asleep, it was as if we had been infused with a medicine that conferred eternal immunity against fear and loneliness and all the dangers of the world.

Chapter 11

Loaded down with toys from Schwarz's and trinkets from Abercrombie's, we flew back to Washington, Sandy thinking of her new black fur coat and I, Cassandra-like, certain we were headed toward disaster. Sandy's appointment book for the days before Christmas reads like a double exposure of a soft, snowy mountain scene and a forest fire:

> *Saturday, December 17:*
>> Doctor
>> Dinner here
>> Buddy here
>> Concert: Joan Sutherland
> *Sunday, December 18:*
>> Mr. Brand to fix furniture
>> Church: Lovely lessons and carol service
>> Neighbors: party at our house

Christmas tree cutting party
Crisis

Tuesday, December 20:

Photo Supply regarding Christmas photos
Ridgewell's here with punch bowl, etc.
Pick up descant book, St. John's Church
Bryn Mawr club luncheon to hear four scholarship students
Carol party, 8:30, here. Amelia here to help
Grand success

Thursday, December 22:

Go by Saville Bookshop to take care of Arnold Lear's present
Collect for Children's Hospital
Doctor: Gloria to take baby
Diana and Taylor Walker here for lunch
Pack for Boston
Our Christmas, here

Friday, December 23:

Pick up embroidery
Deliver cookies, etc., to cleaners, Scheele's Market, Garbage and Trash Men, hairdresser, Morgan's Pharmacy
Doctor: Transfusion
Le Provençal, SLW, our lunch
Coming out party. Dinner before; dance, Mayflower

Saturday, December 24:

Call Buddy about blood tests
Fly Boston: Eastern Number 130, Leave 12:25 Arrive 1:37

Even though her appointment book describes plans for our Christmas carol party, lunches and Christmas preparations, Sandy had to spend all of her afternoons in bed trying to regain some energy. Then she had difficulty sleeping at night and waked up at 4:00 A.M. with her body and thoughts charged to bursting by Prednisone. Rather than lie in bed thrashing and twisting uncomfortably, she put on her wrapper and went down to the kitchen to bake honey or oatmeal bread in the dark, returning to my side before dawn. She complained to her doctors about the ravages from the high doses of medicine and expressed puzzled despair about continuing to be sick for so long.

The carol party, begun the year we were married, was now a large one and included European carols — Swedish, Russian, and Norwegian — sung by friends from those countries. A number of us joined in playing the Bach Fifth Brandenburg Concerto as a finale.

During this time Sandy went through another leukemic crisis; her hemoglobin level plummeted to 5 grams and she had to endure increased dosages of drugs and hour upon hour on the transfusion table.

Because of the carol party and leaving for Boston on Christmas Eve, we had to have "our

Christmas" with Gloria in Washington on the twenty-second of December. For the first time in our own house and with our own little child, we exchanged gifts and celebrated the great event of Christ's birth.

Sandy decided to get Arnold Lear an especially handsome two-volume edition of *Painting in the National Gallery in Washington* and scurried around to buy that and lots of other presents for children, helpers and friends.

On Friday, December twenty-third, I talked with Arnold Lear and Buddy about the proposed trip to Boston. Medically, it was a bad idea, as Sandy's peripheral blood had lots of blasts in it, her energy was low, and the methotrexate was no longer effective. Arnold said she shouldn't go to Boston because of the energy the trip would use up and the difficulty of supervising her care, especially if she needed a transfusion. Buddy reluctantly agreed to the trip, noting that Sandy could see a hematology consultant in Boston, for he was eager that her parents have the comfort of a corroborative consultation with a famous hematologist in Boston.

We had quite a hot session, as I was becoming irritable about having to plan for a transfusion in Boston, hospitalization there if necessary, special

personnel to meet us with a wheelchair at both airports and the general hopelessness of the entire en-
terprise, especially since it had been my idea.

I wanted desperately for us to clear this last
great hurdle. If we could make it, see Sandy's family and have a happy Christmas together, there
would be nothing left to be done. The ringing
doorbell at 3018 N Street was a bother, especially
when it announced the arrival of Ridgewell's with
gold chairs and a punch bowl for the Christmas
carol party, a man with a new dress for Sandy, or
the presence of Mr. Brand, a furniture restorer,
who was fixing our chairs for the future. No future
existed, so I thought, and I sometimes wanted to
hit out in complaint and bewilderment. But I was
wrong, as one always is when he thinks that no future exists.

At the end of our discussion the doctors agreed
to our travel plans. However, they decided Sandy
needed a transfusion before going, very much as
one fills up an automobile with a tank of gas before
a trip. Buddy, Arnold and I discussed the handling
of complications in Boston in case she was not able
to return to Washington, even the possibility that
she might die there. We left each other with sad
handshakes and gravely stated wishes for a Merry
Christmas and a good New Year.

Sandy had her transfusion while I delivered Christmas presents to friends. Because the transfusion continued until 1:30 P.M. we met at Buddy's office and left from there for our special Christmas lunch.

We went to what was then a new and good French restaurant in Washington, Le Provençal. Both of us ordered Punt e Mes, clicked our glasses, and were drinking to our good fortune in being able to wangle the trip from the doctors, when the door to Le Provençal opened and in trooped Buddy, Arnold Lear, Jack Rheingold and Ed Adelson. They were having their own Christmas lunch celebration. These four devoted doctors, easily as distinguished as the "four doctors" in the Sargent painting, took one single afternoon a year to be together and cleanse themselves of heart attacks, blood chemistries, leukemia and tuberculosis. They were startled on coming in the door of the restaurant to see Sandy and me holding hands at our table and chattering away about Christmas plans.

Buddy came up first, kissed Sandy, and wished us a second happy Christmas. He asked about our plans for flying to Boston, trying to control his surprise and uncertainty at finding us out in a restaurant after the transfusion and our serious talk that

morning. Jack, Ed and Arnold came up and we exchanged further happy greetings. I said something
about hoping Sandy's drink wouldn't dilute the
good blood cells she had gotten that morning, and
Sandy wished them all a happy holiday, thanked
them for making it possible for her to go to Boston,
and had me order a bottle of champagne for them.

With a heavy snowstorm impeding our depar-
ture, we pointed toward Boston for our true
Christmas with Sandy's family. Sandy cradled Russell in her lap at the airport as we sat and waited
for the weather to open up. Cutting through a blur
of gray-white snow, ours was the last plane to fly
out of Washington that Christmas holiday. The
Eastern Airlines flight attendant told me the airport was being closed down after the Boston plane
left the gate. We were met in Boston by Miss
Znamiecki, an Eastern Airlines service representa-
tive who became part of our lives from then on,
smoothing the way in and out of wheelchairs, waiting lounges and cars.

We had a long and splendid Christmastime with
all of Sandy's family gathered around. By that time
life had become a bit unreal and for weeks afterwards it seemed that a kind of play was going on.
The largest family gathering in years brought

Sandy's relatives together under a great Christmas tree for eggnog and champagne, toasts and carols on Christmas Eve.

One cold day Sandy and I had lunch at the top of the new Prudential Tower, and afterward walked gaily along Tremont Street and Copley Square, giddy from wine and nipped by the sharp wind. But other times during the holiday Sandy needed long afternoon rests, sat very quietly by my side in the evening, and had to be helped upstairs to bed. At a dinner party with twenty-six assorted adults and children, lots of wine and pleasing talk, and Sandy the center of conversation and interest, it was still a family gathering, not unlike many Saturday night turkey dinners on Cape Cod. Perhaps it was the ability to make small talk and ask about friends in Washington and plans for the spring that got everyone through with warmth and ease. Not a word passed between her father and me about Sandy's condition, but the amount of unstated feeling was immense.

On the last day of the year Sandy kissed all of her family good-bye, gave special hugs to her mother and father, and, laden with a steam shovel and a hobbyhorse for Russell, we were driven to the airport by her brother Harry. Once again attended by Eastern Airlines' Miss Znamiecki, who bundled Sandy into a wheelchair and allowed Russell, Sandy, Niccolo and me to luxuriate in the VIP lounge as we waited for the Washington plane, we settled into that difficult period, the return from vacation.

One more milestone had passed, in many ways the major one. Sandy had seen her family all together for a final time. I had honestly not expected that she would make it through this period, and my relief was great. I had no further plans now and wondered on the plane, as Russell bounced from one of my knees to the other, whatever was going to happen to him.

Back in Washington we had the new year to consider. I looked to it bleakly. But Sandy already had planned for a house-party weekend in the country.

Chapter 12

Even though Sandy and I fell in love at a certain moment during a formal, intown New Year's Eve party, we often talked of having New Year's celebrations in the country, away from dancing and parties. Our vision was the one of Floria Tosca and Mario Cavaradossi in Puccini's *Tosca*; we hoped to escape to the country, where life would be harmonious and simple. Ella Burling's place on the Eastern Shore of Maryland gave us this opportunity. The house was a haven and protection, and all the land around reflected peace. The long fields stretched far into the stands of swaying pines. Snow covered the park, folding over the small hills leading down to the Chesapeake Bay. Flocks of Canadian geese honked and flew freely overhead, safe now that the hunters were gone.

Sandy invited some old friends, Wendy and Roger Cortesi with their baby daughter Tina to come for the New Year weekend. They arrived in characteristic high spirits and with lots of champagne. We showed them the great house — the servants' rooms behind the immense kitchen with its three stoves, the view of the Bay from Ella Burling's bedroom, the little chapel adjoining the house. The chapel, a remnant of pre–Civil War days, contained four pews and a tiny altar surmounted by a Christus sinuously draped over the cross. We stopped there for a moment, perplexed, and then went on to walk through the cornfields and toward the water. On our first exploration of the place I had been delighted to find the chapel and thought of it as a kind of good omen, but I went there rarely, and Sandy, too, stayed away from it. Maybe we felt that prayer was not our path.

We sat before the fire a bit, watched Russell and Tina roll around on the floor, and planned our New Year's Eve supper.

Early in the afternoon I called Mr. Otis Jones at the general store to ask if he could get some oysters. In this magical store it was not necessary for Otis to call a supplier in Baltimore two days before and order the oysters he would need for the next week, packed in ice and getting increasingly stale and tasteless. It was all much simpler in Claiborne. Otis merely had to turn from his telephone to the men huddled around his stove and say, "Arem, you feel like going out and raking up some oysters for the doctor?" And Arem or someone else who had the interest and courage would challenge the gray, damp coldness of the afternoon, get in his boat, and row out a few hundred yards, where he would rake up six dozen oysters quickly, bring them back, clean them, open them, and bring them to our door, more than enough for the afternoon and an oyster stew the next evening. Along with the oysters we got salty stories about how cold it was on the Bay and recollections of what oystering had been like back in the "old days."

That evening we sat around a crackling fire and squeezed lemon juice on the oysters before gulping them down with Chablis.

On a warm Washington evening, two years before, Roger and Wendy had joined us with two other friends to squeeze lemon juice over an entire kilogram of fresh, large, gray-white, soft pearls of Persian caviar. I had just come back from a Peace Corps working assignment to Pakistan and Iran, and my last act in Iran was to buy a kilo of delicious caviar at a ridiculously small price. As soon as

I returned to Washington we arranged for a little party out in our garden to enjoy the special fruits of the trip. We drank champagne, squeezed lemon juice over the caviar, and became quite intoxicated with everything. After all of our gorging, we adjourned to the house and sang arias from *Don Giovanni*. We had a hilarious time singing, playing the flute, and mimicking the various missing bass, soprano and tenor parts. And so, squeezing lemon juice over the wet, slippery salty oysters before we downed them in one swallow reminded us of another happy time, but a more hopeful and even innocent time.

After consuming all the oysters and Chablis, we walked through the cold hallway to Ella Burling's high-ceilinged austere dining room, dominated by a long, narrow refectory table. When first married, along with the simple joys of loving each other, playing tennis, and holding hands, Sandy and I talked occasionally about furniture. One of her greatest wishes was to have a fifteenth-century Italian refectory table. We now had one, courtesy of Ella Burling, graced by Sandy and Wendy in long dresses, like sparkling jewels in the candlelight. Even though Sandy's face and stomach had become puffy and were out of proportion to the slimness of her legs and arms, her radiance warmed the night. Before sitting down to the dinner she had quietly gone to the kitchen to take her heavy evening dose of Prednisone.

Talk of the Washington Opera Society at dinner turned us to reminiscing about Washington's happiest party, called The Dancing Class, which was presided over by Roger's aunt and uncle, who were also powers in the Opera Society. Roger's aunt, an old friend of Sandy's parents, showed almost unprecedented kindness by allowing Sandy and me to rejoin The Dancing Class as a couple soon after our marriage. Usually, single people, upon marriage, were stricken from the guest list, and had to wait years to be reinvited as a couple. We joked about that being the reason so many Washington bachelors remained that way — they didn't want to forfeit their invitations to The Dancing Class parties, where Meyer Davis's exuberant band played bouncy tunes and the champagne flow was continuous.

Full of wine and happiness, we settled back in the deep, soft chairs of the living room before the fire. Midnight and the New Year came quietly and we drank to our children, with Roger adding a toast to "more champagne and caviar this year."

Sandy and Wendy faded quickly, probably because Roger and I were becoming rather foolishly giddy. After they went upstairs to bed Roger and I sat with cigars, blowing smoke in the air toward the high ceiling of the room.

"Sidney, my good man," Roger said, "we have more champagne. Let's drink it." I had always admired Roger's great, ranging knowledge of biology, psychiatry, psychoanalysis, science in general, literary figures, Italian opera arias, and his prodigious ability to drink. When we went to his house for dinner, even though there were only six or eight people, four or five bottles of wine would be consumed. He lived up to my admiration this New Year's morning. After chaffing me a bit about the impending take-over of psychiatry by biology, Roger, in his slightly stammering, quick voice, blurted out, "Why is Sandy's face so puffy, Sidney?" He sat back, adjusted his glasses, and blew smoke in the air, waiting expectantly.

"It's an anemia, Roger," I said.

"What kind of anemia?" he asked slowly. Roger was never satisfied with incomplete answers, and he sensed that I wanted to tell him more. I wanted desperately to share what I knew with him and the champagne helped me to do so.

"Please keep this between us," I said. "Sandy

doesn't know the diagnosis. I've spoken about it only to her brothers in Boston and a few people here. Sandy has leukemia."

He looked away. "I wondered about that." Then, "But they can do something? She will get better?"

I drank some champagne and stared at the fire. "Roger, she may live for a while, but she won't get better. There is always a chance, of course, but acute granulocytic leukemia just doesn't get better."

"But she'll live for a long time?"

"Her doctors have always said maybe a few days, maybe a few months," I answered.

"Oh, Sidney, my friend —" He reached for more champagne. "You mean she is going to die, Sandy is going to die?"

We both cried. He got up, lit his cigar, and then sat down and put his arms around my shoulders. He is the only American man I know who can hug and embrace another man.

"Sidney, you can't mean it."

We opened another bottle and I told him of the months after the christening at which he had been godfather, of the transfusions, her bravery, of the utter hopelessness of it all. "Oh, Sidney, Sidney," he repeated, "not Sandy." Before going to bed we finished a fourth bottle of champagne. Roger, unable to be helpful medically as Buddy was, less articulate than Les Glenn, but more my contemporary, was the third of four people to be of great help to me. Finally, we crawled upstairs to our beds, he to Wendy and I to clamber unsteadily into bed beside Sandy, brush her cheek with a kiss, and fall into oblivion.

The next morning was terrible. Rainy weather, champagne fumes and cigar smoke everywhere. Roger and I were a bit sheepish about our feelings of the night before, and I was incredibly unsteady through the day. But Sandy and Wendy and Russell and Tina were full of good spirits and thought we were only victims of our own gluttony. Maybe we were. We packed up Russell, clothes, medicines and bundled ourselves back to the new year in Washington.

Chapter 13

 Sandy taught French to fifth-grade
boys at the Potomac School in Virginia the rest of the year, though she
found it increasingly difficult to get
there regularly and her appointment book increasingly records more missed classes. A good deal of
our dinner conversation consisted of "Darling,
those hoodlums in my morning class just will *not*
learn French. Godfrey's Tweezers, they really get
me down when they talk and are inattentive. One
of them just can't get the idea. And his head looks
deformed to me."

I would laugh and try to give sage child psychiatry advice, but my suggestions rarely worked and
we puzzled over two particular boys in the class
many times. Sandy stuck at it, and the boys con-

tinued to be resolutely poor French students for all the months left.

As a direct consequence of our trip to New York Sandy made an appointment with Dr. Hazen Shea in mid-January. Dr. Shea is the obstetrician who brought Russell out into the world squalling and squinting on a hot, muggy May sixteenth the year before. At Russell's birth the spinal anesthesia wore off early and Hazen had to pull him out with forceps, leaving a temporary contusion and a permanent, rather handsome birthmark. Sandy experienced a lot of pain with this unanticipated natural childbirth. I had suggested natural childbirth but she, not a "modern" woman nor interested in innovations, wanted things done the usual way. Despite the pain, Sandy had recovered enough to call her mother in Boston a half hour after Russell was born. Through a mist of Demerol and weakness she announced with pleasure over the telephone, "I've given my husband a baby boy," and then broke down in tears on my shoulder.

She was in high spirits by the evening and I smuggled some champagne into the hospital to toast our happiness. Flouting convention, Sandy protested that she felt too well to stay in the hospital and decided to go home after three days. Dr.

Shea agreed and we had a grand procession to our house with Sandy, baby, nurse, Niccolo and flowers. She was overjoyed to be in her own house again, to sleep under her own pale blue silk bed-cover on a linen pillow slip, to have all of her powders, brushes and various ointments spread out on the table in our bedroom, and most important, to have Russell gurgling in the next room, surrounded by his tiny crib, a bassinet, a little pine chest and a white rocker.

The day after Sandy returned home a few friends came in the afternoon for a visit. I excused myself after bringing them upstairs to gather around Sandy as she cradled Russell in her arms, and hurried down where two musician friends were waiting to join me in springing a surprise. I had transcribed the great anthem from *The Messiah*, "For unto us a child is born, unto us a son is given," for the unlikely combination of two flutes and a violin. While everyone was chattering upstairs, I got my flute and joined the other musicians in playing that ineffably lovely theme and later the high, thrilling descant that follows. Afterward we all gathered for champagne around Sandy's bed. Those were the glad tidings of Russell's birth.

This time Sandy went to see Dr. Shea because

her abdomen was enlarging and her breasts tingled. Since she was taking such a mass of medicines it was impossible to know whether and when she might have another menstrual period, and we had made love in New York at the beginning of December. Dr. Shea examined her and took urine for a pregnancy test, which he reported as negative. Though we very much wanted another child, and I particularly wanted a daughter, I realized that the days of our rejoicing in a pregnancy were over forever, and we were both pleased at the result of the examination. But it left us puzzled, because Sandy was having some pain in her abdomen and was reacting oddly to the Prednisone.

It was most puzzling. Sandy had all the signs of pregnancy, but the test was negative. Her body was beginning to come apart in some ways; in others it was strong. Her gums bled almost all the time after she brushed her teeth; small black-and-blue blotches appeared on her skin; she experienced fleeting pain in her pelvis and lower back; and her hemoglobin level continued to drop, despite transfusions. Yet the blast cells, the ominous leukemia cells, disappeared from her bloodstream and she was, most of the time, fresh with energy and plans.

Was this a remission or a silent, enigmatic sign of disintegration?

During this post-Christmas period we became exasperated with each other a number of times over such weighty issues as diapering Russell, and a houseguest who, in my opinion, stayed too long. Also, Sandy became irritated with people in Georgetown. She returned from the grocery store one day, slammed the garden door, livid with anger, and exclaimed, "Fred Scheele said I looked like a chipmunk!" She insisted that I go immediately and tell him the reason that her cheeks were swollen was that she was taking a lot of powerful medicine for her anemia. Ordinarily, she was the last person to be angry at anyone for anything. But now she was adamant and demanded that I speak with Fred. I trudged over to his market on Dumbarton Avenue and gave him a rather odd explanation for Sandy's situation. Naturally, he said that he'd been joking and that he would apologize to her when he saw her next. Her reaction reflected the power of cortisone and other medication to put her on edge, as well as a new vulnerability she felt about her beauty, which she had for so long taken for granted. As a calming joke I painted a large sign reading:

PROCLAMATION

By unbiased unanimous vote the following person
is acclaimed

THE MOST EXCITING, DESIRABLE,
RARE AND BEAUTIFUL GIRL
IN ALL THE WORLD
— *ALEXANDRA WERKMAN* —

Judges: (All experienced men about town)
Russell Werkman
Niccolo
Sidney Werkman

The proclamation was decorated with a scrawl
made by Russell as I held his hand, and a paw
print by Niccolo. Sandy dismissed the episode
lightly, but hung the sign on the bedroom wall and
never took it down.

Other quarrels followed and we decided to get
away from Washington for a short time to help
quiet ourselves down. Because we had been happy
before at Boca Grande, a lovely, long spit of land
on the warm west coast of Florida, which was also
close to good medical facilities and an airport in
Sarasota, we bustled about, making plans to fly
there.

Despite her enlarging abdomen, pain, occasional bleeding and the feeling that a mass was growing inside her, Sandy rushed around from Lord and Taylor's to Saks, buying clothes, preparing for Russell's stay in Washington with her mother and father, who came down from Boston to baby-sit, arranging dinner parties for them, and planning our own trip. She arranged for Mlle. Pallu, who had been Russell's nurse on the Cape the previous summer, to come and help Gloria during the time we were away in the sun. Before leaving on a Saturday, Sandy popped into Arnold Lear's office, almost as if she were getting a typhoid fever shot before going overseas, to have a last transfusion of two pints of packed red blood cells.

Boca Grande was a tonic for both of us. Our room in the Gasparilla Inn looked out on the lagoon and palm trees and the long green swath of golf course. The sunny, placid days swept by with swimming, looking for seashells in one of the finest hunting places in the world, deep-sea fishing, and all the other delights of the seashore. Sandy tried bicycling but tired quickly. Her element was the water and she exulted in it and was renewed.

At Boca Grande she informed anyone who would listen that she was off two more pills, making it easier for her to think, sleep, and get around in general. From this time on, she became wrapped up increasingly in her illness and her attempt to fight it. She thought that exercise was the key, as far back as our last tennis game in October. And at that time, though I knew only too well what the future held, we had played the tennis. Now, hoping to keep some remnant of a former reality in such a changed life, I encouraged her perilous wish to exercise as much as she wanted.

A former captain of the Bryn Mawr College swimming team, Sandy looked out at the great expanse of the Florida gulf water and hit on the idea of swimming twenty laps every day. She planned a course for herself and was exceedingly proud to make the distances set each day. I watched her from a beach chair and wondered what sort of fish was this that could swim so well but was doomed to drown. She would come out of the water, hair dripping down her shoulders, and say, "I did more laps today than yesterday. I'm sure I'm getting better."

"I know you are," I replied.

Then Sandy would plead, "Won't you call Arnold and ask him if I can be taken off another pill? I know these pills are causing a lot of my trouble. I feel so good now." I always nodded and spoke of talking with Arnold when we returned to Washington.

We spent a lot of time on lazy afternoons in Boca Grande reading books from the Furst Library. Over a Punt e Mes before dinner we made plans for the summer. Sandy liked our waitress very much and contracted for her to come to the Cape for the summer to help out at her family's house. I sat there befuddled at the incredible confidence, even exuberance, she showed.

We saw omens in remarkable shells along the beach, talks with people who worked both at Boca Grande and at other summer places we knew, friends we chanced upon who had been in weddings with us years ago — all kinds of happy coincidences. In our search of the remarkable Furst Library, I looked for books that spoke of strength and courage and all the other consummate ideals. There and everywhere the books fell far short of my hopes. The person who endowed the library, Johann Furst, had written a book called *Triumph Over Pain*, but it contained more philosophy than triumph.

Sandy had periods of lethargy, when she was disappointed that she couldn't be completely herself. Her lack of energy on a bicycle disturbed her, and I quickly returned the bicycles to keep her from fretting. She tanned well in the tropical sun, too well because of the Prednisone she was taking. Though her cheeks remained puffy, she was pleased to note that she was getting bosomy again. We didn't know whether the padding was the result of the medicine or pregnancy, but Sandy rather proudly bought a bigger, looser bathing suit to encase her enlarging breasts and abdomen.

It was another honeymoon. We became fresh, free spirits exploring each other, proud of the simplest things — catching a fish, taking a picture, and planning to display the shells we picked up on the long, wet beach.

Early morning was a special time. We would awake with the sun and turn to each other with murmurs of yawning delight. From the time of our first weekends together at Cape Cod, at Martha's Vineyard, or in little inns on the Eastern Shore of Maryland, as we each defined ourselves to each other in small preferences, particular desires, Sandy showed her love of the dawn, and my love of it was renewed because of her. Both of us liked to leave curtains open so the sun could flow in at dawn and gently nuzzle us awake. Lying lazily in bed in each other's arms every morning, we had outside our window the long flat, almost Dutch, vista down to the Boca Grande lagoon as the sun rose through the clumps of palm trees.

But one morning Sandy interrupted our caressing. "Darling, it hurts," she said. We were silent a few moments and then I asked her how it hurt, hoping it was only some kind of inflammation or infection, like the one she had had on a winter holiday in Jamaica several years before. I wasn't so blind as I had been in September when we played tennis and had ignored the black-and-blue marks on her legs. I guessed that it was a leukemic infiltration, but reminded Sandy of Jamaica and our technical problems in making love down there.

"Maybe your insides just don't like to make love in idyllic places," I explained wryly, and she was somewhat reassured, but we began to want to get home and see Dr. Shea again.

One evening we drove from the main part of Boca Grande to visit friends, Mr. and Mrs. MacLaren, who managed a large, old prisonlike hotel on the outskirts of the town. We sat at their dark bar and had daiquiris as Sandy and Mrs. MacLaren engaged in deep conversation. Sandy spoke about her anemia, Russell's birth and our life in Washington. Then Mrs. MacLaren began a long discussion of the thyroid tumor which had been removed from her neck that year.

"I'm just blessed to be here," she said. She described in detail the operation and its results and her happy feeling of deliverance from a malignancy that might have killed her. Mr. MacLaren scrubbed the bar vigorously, as he realized we were not going to be allowed to pay our bill for drinks. In that decrepit hotel the question of payment was important, as they had absolutely no guests at the time. It was a marvelous hotel with a great lobby going right to the sky and tropical plants growing in the center of it. All of us drank too much, and as we left, Mrs. MacLaren gave Sandy a great hug. Then she took off the red coral necklace she was wearing and pressed it in Sandy's hand. Sandy tried to give it back, but Mrs. MacLaren wouldn't let her. "It will be good luck for your anemia," she said. "It will charm all the bad spirits away and protect you."

After great embraces all around we walked out of the hotel, promising we would return to visit next year. We drove our rented car to the end of the road toward the sea and sat, heads and shoulders together, holding hands, looking out at the moon and stars. I knew Sandy was happy, and we had never been so much in love.

After a long silence Sandy murmured, "Darling, I'm going to give you a big fortieth birthday party this May. We'll find out when Howard Devron is free so his band can play, and we'll put up a tent in the garden. I'll have Mrs. Karthy bake your favorite cookies, and we'll just have champagne, cookies, and steak tartare."

"Great," I said, but with a sinking feeling thought to myself, "She thinks she's going to live that long." I could picture it. We would make all the plans and then the day before the party she would have a relapse and we would have to let the party go on while she was upstairs in bed dying. With an effort I kidded her about advertising my age, especially as we had seen one of her old boyfriends at Boca Grande.

On our way back to Washington we stopped in one of the Sarasota Keys to visit with Mr. David Grey, a ninety-one-year-old friend of Sandy's. Sandy and he remembered each other warmly from summers on Cape Cod. Mr. Grey's mind was still nimble and twinkly, though his body was crippled by age. Obviously, Sandy had charmed him years ago, and he was still enchanted by her and she by him.

He told us of his belief in a faith healer who helped him with his arthritis and low back pain. Sandy was eager to hear about this. Mr. Grey gave us lunch and talked about his remarkable conversion to Christian Science. They were like conspirators, discussing their symptoms, each eagerly hoping that the faith healer would be useful to the other. Sandy debated staying down an extra day in order to meet this extraordinary healer. Even I wavered but then reminded her of how much we missed Russell, and she quickly agreed to give up the healer. Laden with bags of grapefruit, oranges and seashells, we flew back to Washington, to the other world we inhabited.

Chapter 14

Winter in Washington limped on through parties, care of the baby and walks around Georgetown. Sandy had periods of weakness and glum spirits, then perked up and taught her French classes at Potomac School, joined a swimming group, and planned for the future. The transfusions continued, each one entailing a day lost in the half-dark recesses of a little room, where Sandy idled out the hours lying on a narrow bed. Afterward she felt buoyant for a time but then fell back into lethargy. And in the late winter a repeat pregnancy test done by Dr. Shea came back positive.

We had both suspected she was pregnant after our New York idyll, but the tests had been negative. However, her body was changing in that happy pregnant way, and I always felt that the lilt

and energy Sandy possessed in January were due
to the early changes of pregnancy. Naturally, we
wanted more children but this was no time for another. Sandy, Dr. Shea and I agreed, almost without discussion, that an abortion had to be done.
Brief consideration of the possibilities — a mal-
formed baby, a dead mother — was enough to
make up our minds. But we had to wait for the
time that would be best medically to do the abortion. And when that time came, we had to wait,
like everyone else in this era of overcrowded hospitals, for a bed to be available in the George Washington Hospital.

As spring announced itself with crocuses and
birdsongs, we marked time and waited. An early
Easter was coming, but the thought of it was no
great help.

One morning Sandy proclaimed, "I think I'll go
to Boston for the Chilton Club show. Ellen and
Lisa are both in it, and it will give me a chance to
feel better." She packed carefully and bought
some trinket presents on Wisconsin Avenue to take
with her on the trip to see the annual show at her
mother's club. We drove the familiar curved way
around the Lincoln Memorial and the Pentagon to
the airport. I was almost beginning to hope that
plane trips, for Sandy or me, would finish up life

for us. Every time I flew to places like Manitoba or Detroit to make speeches, a tiny part of me light-heartedly contemplated going up in the plane and never coming down. I wonder if that thought ever crossed Sandy's mind. Probably not, for she simply wasn't made that way.

During her short visit to Boston Sandy had more trouble with bleeding. She phoned me about it and I called Dr. Shea. Suppose she couldn't get back from Boston and all the plans and medical care had to be changed to that town? We had waited for a hospital in Washington for days and now we were in danger of having to hospitalize her in a medically strange town. It was like the dread of having a skiing accident in Sestriere or Gstaad instead of Aspen. And time was becoming a factor. The little clock ticking in Sandy's uterus was becoming a larger fetus. The great dictum that abortions have to be done before a pregnancy is three months in process was catching up with us.

From medical and personal experience I knew only too well the feeling of ominous anxiety one had when waiting for an abortion to be organized. There is the great problem of life itself — we spend a great part of our youth loving and worrying about pregnancy, then want that very pregnancy more than anything in the world. To end a life with an abortion is absurd. Sandy's trip to Boston seemed to underscore the whole foolishness of life and made me feel, as I did so many times, a helpless futility — like the partisan soldier in an Italian World War II movie about Venice who had no ammunition left for his carbine and knew he was a sitting duck for the Nazis approaching in the near distance along the flat salt marshes outside Venice.

Fortunately Sandy was able to fly back to Washington and we were told a room would be available at the hospital in three days.

Sandy collapsed on the big silk chair in our bedroom, weary, and yet relieved to go to the hospital at last. "Gloria," she called in her high, quavering voice, "would you please come in and help me rummage through some of these bed things? I'll need some nighties and my silk wrapper for that awful hospital." Gloria opened Sandy's red suitcase and put in all the paraphernalia of traveling — toothbrush, hairbrush, slippers, clock, hairpins, handkerchiefs, underwear.

Sandy left lists for Scheele's Market, the cleaners, notes for Mr. Brand, who was coming to repair the legs of some furniture, and organized Mlle. Pallu so Gloria could have a day free. The last night we had a quiet dinner and discussed details for the fortieth birthday party — the musicians, tent, barmen and glasses. Then she was on the phone with friends, arranging dinner parties before the dance.

The next morning Sandy checked into the hospital for the first time, the signal of an ominous change in our lives. In the emergency room several of the medical students I taught were there to wish us well. When we got to the ward, blood was drawn by a medical student I knew and the first history was taken, by one of my students. I was proud of these students and their demeanor with Sandy — shy, yet competent, warm and decent. She always liked them and answered their questions as if they were professors.

All of Sandy's doctors converged in the dark hallways of ward South 3, a place filled incongruously with flowers and bedpans, wheelchairs, and white-coated interns writing histories. Sandy's room, with its straight white bed and plastic chairs, its TV set staring down obliquely from the ceiling, looked like part of a sterile, grotesque motel.

Many times in the past we had driven miles to find quiet little inns where we could be alone and unobserved by the world, but here her room was open for all to see or walk in, the human body, with all its secrets displayed, in the pathetic hope that something could be done for it. Except this time there was no hope. It was all illusion, all watching a clock that had stopped, a football play when the game is over. Does the halfback who drops the end-zone pass in a Rose Bowl game re-play that one over and over and over again? Is there no way to recapture and change the past? We are so oblivious to the finality of a moment that we have lived intently. We seldom recognize what a pinnacle it is to love and be safe. All we know is that life contains so many years to eke out after the great events are over. These were some of the thoughts I mooned over, standing beside Sandy's hospital bed.

Sandy rarely philosophized. She lived and tried to give pleasure and a measure of orderliness to life, a kind of form in the present.

People came in. Students to draw blood, with their syringe, cotton swab, rubber tourniquet. An aide left a bottle for urinalysis. All the body fluids that are kept so secret from the world most of the time, and some that are secret from the person himself except for a cut finger that bleeds, are exposed in the hospital.

Sandy lay on her bed, blood dripping into her left arm. She was given an enema before the abortion was started, as if anything very much could be left in her body. She sucked cracked ice to moisten her parched lips and I wiped them with glycerine, smoothed her hair, and tried to talk of pleasant things.

"We'll get some yellow ribbon and Easter eggs for Russell. And I'll ask Wendy and Roger to come over Sunday for breakfast and an Easter egg hunt. Then we'll come to visit you here and maybe they'll spring you by Monday." I drawled on, bemused, with Sandy holding my hand, both of us staring at the millions of platelets trickling into her forearm.

The bag of sticky red-brown blood hanging like a flag from its holder dominated the white hospital room. It looked like a transparent hot-water bottle, but it was more a cocktail shaker, for it contained, not only the precious blood and its platelets, but also an antihistamine to prevent an allergic fever reaction that could kill Sandy by pushing her temperature beyond its present 104° level, and an antibiotic to hold in check any infections that might be introduced by the abortion. The antibiotic was crucial because all human beings are host to hundreds of millions of bacteria. Ordinarily, the bacteria live benignly in our guts and mouths and ears and on our skin. But in a sense, they lie in wait for the time when the body is weak and then they become as powerful and malignant as cholera or plague or meningitis. They overwhelm the body through the bloodstream, depleting the white blood cells that try to fight them and defeating the other body defenses of hormones and proteins and phagocytes.

These bacteria were feared by Hazen Shea as he measured the distance between Sandy's umbilicus and the symphysis pubis bone in the pelvis, palpated the top of her uterus through the skin and muscle of her abdomen, and prepared his immense syringe and needle. The syringe contained salt solution which would be injected into the uterus to stir up its contents and extrude them into the world of living things.

The classical method of abortion is to scrape the inside of the uterine cavity with a small knife or curette, as much to stir the uterus to begin to contract rhythmically as in the hope that a small instrument can locate an even smaller egg in a vast, almost empty space. Whether done with a stone implement or a gleaming, graceful curette under impeccable conditions, the procedure is a simple one and quickly completed. Its major problems are technical. The surgeon doing the abortion must be certain that he does not pierce the uterus, his operating technique must be absolutely sterile so that

135

he does not introduce infection, and he must understand the use of hormones so he can give the patient adequate medication to stop bleeding and make the uterus contract after the baby is born. It is ironic that, though the operation is not complicated, countless babies, unwanted, maimed, have wandered through life because an abortion was not available to their mothers.

Until recently only one reliable method of abortion was known. Then the novel idea of injecting saline into the uterine cavity to stimulate the beginning of contraction and the natural process of ejection was thought of. It offered a valuable alternative treatment for women who cannot tolerate much bleeding from curetting or the possibility of developing infection.

Sandy was in just that position. Either bleeding or infection would finish her, so we were blessed to be able to call upon another procedure. Also, with the injection technique she did not need to be anesthetized, sparing her system another terrible danger. But she did need to go through the contractions. After Hazen put in the saline, we waited all afternoon for something to happen.

"The only thing that's happened is my tummy hurts and my fever has stayed up," Sandy said. We waited. I tried to read to her from Lawrence Durrell's *Stiff Upper Lip*, but it didn't seem funny to her. She tried needlepoint but was too tired and weak for cross-stitching.

"We have to get the garden started on time this year," Sandy said, holding her unfinished carnation needlepoint pattern up to the light to inspect it. "I'm going to call Katy Keck. She knows all about flowers. And I want to get some big concrete vases to place around near the garden gate." She talked about the need for more furniture and about the birthday party in May. That party was beginning to get my goat. I was preoccupied with all the possible ways Sandy could die before morning and the thought of ordering champagne, glasses and chairs from Ridgewell's was too much for me to handle.

Hazen Shea and Buddy stayed on into the evening and I drove home for a few hours to play with Russell before he went to sleep. When I returned Sandy's fever was inching up beyond 105° and she was restless, full of pain and generally unhappy. Buddy walked me out to my car, when it was clear that I was worse than useless in the hospital. We sat in the front seat, looking through the windshield at the equestrian statue of George Washington in the circle near the hospital.

"What in the world can be done?" I said, after a long silence.

"Nothing now," Buddy answered, shaking his head. "Her temperature is 105°, and we're not keeping up with her in blood. She just doesn't have any immune mechanisms working."

"She may die tonight then," I said, as much to myself as to Buddy, but he answered anyway.

"She may, Sidney."

"What is it like afterward?" I asked gropingly, trying to find words that would look over an abyss. The "afterward" still on my tongue, with some "uh's" and throat clearing, I managed, "I mean . . . I mean . . . do you know anybody who has married again?"

Buddy mentioned the name of another doctor. "He's married again and even has three children with his wife now."

After a long pause I whispered, "Is it the same?"

"It's never the same," Buddy said slowly.

"But does he love his new wife?"

"It's not the same as having a Sandy."

To try to pull back from an impossible vision of the future, I started to tell him how great he had been in every way, but he put his hand on my shoulder and said he had to get back in the hospital to see how a patient with a myocardial infarction was doing.

I switched on the engine and swung off into

138

Washington Circle toward home, wondering if I wanted to remain a doctor if such things had to be told, if the only time illness hit your family, that illness was death.

Hazen stayed until 1 A.M., waiting to see if real contractions would start. Sandy told me later he talked to her about his childhood in Ohio, how his father was mayor of the town where he grew up, and about horses and riding and happy times.

I made a last trip to the hospital that night, but Sandy was dozing. At 3 A.M., when the pain and loneliness increased, she was startled to have the phone in her room ring. It was Buddy. "I just got up to take a phone call from a patient and wanted to know how you were, dear," he said to her.

For the rest of the night Sandy lay dozing and waiting for movement in her belly. Nurses popped in and out. The next day she reported, "These nurses you consort with lead complicated lives. They came and sat at my bed early in the morning and we talked about their love affairs, and they asked about you. One of them had a rotation at Children's Hospital."

Through most of Saturday morning Sandy felt mild contractions. Her fever decreased and remained stable at a lower level. She was not permitted any food because of the danger of vomiting during the delivery. She became hungry but found chewing and sucking on ice a poor substitute for soup or milk.

Finally, as noon passed, the contractions quickened. We wanted that change and dreaded it, for it signaled the crucial moment. When the baby was delivered would Sandy's uterus clamp down and stop the bleeding? If it didn't her doctors would have to try to replace blood as fast as it gushed from her, an impossible task. They had to strike a delicate balance of hormones, pain killers, drugs to stop bleeding, antibiotics, and the continuing Prednisone and methotrexate — all of them potentially working against each other, but necessary just the same.

As if this were not enough, Sandy had the only disagreeable time with a doctor she ever experienced during her illness. An obstetrics resident came in to examine her. He was harsh and heavy-handed when he pushed on her tender abdomen and showed no concern for her cries of complaint. He returned a number of times and treated her roughly on each occasion. Finally, Sandy refused to let him touch her again, saying she was Dr. Shea's patient, not his. He replied that he didn't care whose patient she was, he was going to go ahead with his examination.

Luckily, Buddy came by just then and heard the argument. Furious, he sent the resident from the room and told him not to return. When Buddy, Hazen Shea and the head of obstetrics, who was consulting with Hazen, got together that morning, the obstetrics chief apologized to Sandy for the resident's behavior and assured her he would have it out with him about it.

I cite this incident, even allowing that Sandy may have been tired, irritable, frightened, or groggy from medication, because it was, thankfully, the single ugly moment in over eight months of steady involvement with the medical profession. All the other doctors, nurses, technicians and aides were meticulously capable and far more than simply humanly warm and thoughtful.

Saturday afternoon was gray with patchy rain and mist. Television, the Metropolitan Opera on the radio were of no use. We dawdled the time away wondering whether we were going to have a boy or a girl. As we talked desultorily, Sandy said calmly, "I think it's coming." Hazen Shea put gentle pressure on her abdomen to help the delivery and a little creature about five inches long slid out.

Hazen said, "She's a perfectly formed little girl, Sandy."

Indeed she was, with a lovely, fully formed face

— without the blemishes most babies get from being knocked around in the mother's birth canal during delivery — and all the usual wrinkled pink-brown fingers and toes, but in exquisite miniature, a model of a child that might have been. Sandy wanted to see her and was proud to have given birth to a girl child, even one we couldn't keep.

Though the danger to Sandy's life was still present during these short moments of pleasure, somehow we no longer worried. Hazen had lots of work and sweating to do over how much ergonovine to inject to stanch the bleeding, but Sandy and I dreamed about what to call this little girl. Sandy reminisced about her wish to have been named Anne Hathaway Colt instead of Alexandra, and spoke about her experimentation as a young teen-ager with using that name. Disregarding the anguish of losing our new little baby for a bit we made plans to keep her spirit alive forever and were content the rest of the day.

I walked to a bookstore nearby and got Sandy a volume of the large Skira three-volume *French Painting.* I had given her the first one, on early French paintings, for Russell's birth, and inscribed this one: "A second volume in honor of the series of radiant spirits you have lovingly conceived for us."

On Sunday, Easter morning, all danger was past and recovery was beginning. I carried Russell into the lobby of the hospital and his mother was wheeled down to hold him in her arms. Gloria and I described the yellow and white streamers, colored eggs and an Easter bunny that had appeared mysteriously in our garden that morning, and we shared a chocolate Easter egg in smeary fashion.

No more emergencies marred Sandy's time in the hospital, and I was able to take her home in a week. As the car door closed and I started off from the hospital driveway to our house, Sandy sounded a deserved sour note to me. "Darling," she said, "let's be certain that this kind of thing never, *never* happens again."

Chapter 15

 The abortion left Sandy feeling weak and tired, and both of us needed a respite from Washington and doctors. I promised a trip to Sandy to divert us from the uncertainty about the outcome of her illness, and a visit to Hot Springs, Virginia, had been on our minds for a month, especially during long vigils with pain or when waiting for the last drip of a transfusion.

The trouble was that Sandy's hemoglobin remained very low despite repeated transfusions of packed cells. Also, there were evidences of leukocytic infiltrations in a number of places. The infiltrations showed themselves as tiny balls of raised skin, sometimes no larger than a pinhead, on her back and thighs. The number of small hematomas, swollen areas filled with blood, caused by minor abrasions, increased. It was clear that methotrexate and Prednisone were not doing their jobs. Various changes in medication made no difference. It was like fiddling with a combination lock in a random way. The gain from using methotrexate at the beginning was now being lost, for it had produced its one single brilliant remission and that was all. Not that the other medicines were any more effective, but we knew that this one had finished its job. It meant that Sandy's appeals as to why she was on so much medication and why the medication didn't work could not be answered with any certainty. The main problem was the fear of bleeding and of infection that might follow after bleeding.

We went to see Arnold Lear before going to Hot Springs and had to convince him again that a trip was sensible. I had assured him repeatedly that I would take all responsibility for what might happen, but we went through the discussion yet another time. After blood tests which showed a hemoglobin level of 7 grams, followed by a transfusion of packed cells, Arnold agreed, with many misgivings, that Sandy could make the trip.

There comes a time when medical judgment must bow to another level of judgment, the judgment that tells a doctor to permit a cardiac patient to travel in an airplane, eat forbidden food, or tire

himself out in happy exercise. These decisions —
balancing a full life against merely existing — are
vexing ones in this time of scientific medicine. In
Sandy's case the issues were absolutely clear, for
scientific medicine had little more to offer, but Dr.
Lear knew that the disease had still more tricks to
play on her.

Nevertheless we were elated when Arnold gave
us permission to fly to the Homestead Hotel at Hot
Springs. I had told him I was already familiar with
Hot Springs, from my days as an intern at the University of Virginia Hospital at Charlottesville, before I started psychiatric training.

At that time I was still involved with patients
who had pneumonia, heart attacks or ulcers and
had driven often and happily along the winding,
hilly incline to the Homestead for weekends of re-
cuperation from starting blood transfusions and
palpating hearts and spleens during the long hours
a new doctor spends slaving away in a university
hospital. Being waked up four and five times a
night for emergency calls just as I had taken my
second sock off to fall in bed, left me very tired
during that long year of internship and trips to Hot
Springs had been delightful diversions for me. The
January chill, although no snow was on the ground,
encouraged the pleasures of desultory reading be-

side a big fire and listening to Joe Lanin, the piano player in the hotel, chord out "Cheek to Cheek" and "Mountain Greenery." Joe talked about his famous brothers Lester and Howard, and of how he happened to end up in Hot Springs, while Howard was a well-known bandleader in Philadelphia and Lester a famous one throughout the country. It was blissful to be high in the mountains, far away from patients and share the good conversation of another musician as well as the reminiscences of the courtly old hotel doctor.

While my memories of Hot Springs centered on happy laziness and the welcome respite from starting blood transfusions at Charlottesville, Sandy's were of the stories told her about the healing effect of the medicinal springs on her grandfather and, later, her mother and father, as well as her own recollections of trips she had taken with her parents during spring vacations from school to swim and play tennis.

During the choppy flight down to Hot Springs, Sandy, Russell and Gloria sat on the right-hand side of the plane and I on an aisle seat on the left. Gloria, who had only flown once, from Portugal to Washington, made painfully frightened faces as the plane grazed the treetops of the Blue Ridge Mountains. At one point, when the plane suddenly dropped several hundred feet, Russell leaped out of Sandy's arms to mine and clasped onto me like a monkey for the rest of the flight.

Forced to land in Covington because of high winds, we rented a car there and drove to Hot Springs. Our rooms looked out toward the gentle mountains and the green lawn rolling down to the swimming pool. Arnold Lear promised to keep in close touch while we were away, and I called the doctor at Hot Springs, who was a splendid remnant of a more gracious period in medicine, to prepare him for our coming. I had spent long, lazy times talking with this doctor about water cures, the mineral baths and the special exercising machines from the Skoda Machine Works in Czechoslovakia, never guessing that I would need his help years later for a sick wife.

The mountain air and pleasant atmosphere of the Homestead refreshed us all. After a day of quiet playing in the indoor pool we slept well. Even Russell, only ten months old, loved swimming in the shallow part of the pool. Sandy tried several laps but was too tired to do more. She arranged for a turn in the baths and a massage by the same person who had eased her grandfather's arthritis many years before. The mystique of the hot springs pool and its remarkably curative powers was having its effect, at least on our minds.

The first day at the great Homestead Russell sat at the dinner table with us and showered rolls and forks on the floor, to have them retrieved with great patience by white-gloved waiters. Thereafter we arranged to have his dinner brought to him in his room. It was quite a sight to see an enormous table rolled in, all set for a banquet with silver, flowers, rolls, salt, pepper, condiments neatly arranged on it. With a flourish the waiter would remove the silver cover of Russell's plate to display a tiny hamburger and some chopped carrots.

On the second day, a glorious morning, we got outside in the mountain air early and wheeled Russell around gentle paths in his baby carriage. The sun was warm and the wind rather sharp as we walked along the golf course, crossing several streams. Sandy asked Gloria to wheel Russell's carriage and lagged behind us a bit, though we still chatted about the curling smoke below us in the village and the pine trees swaying easily in the spring air.

"I certainly feel odd," she said.

"Maybe it's the thin air. We're at three thousand feet," I countered, trying to be helpful.

"I don't know what it is, but I'm really tired. I'm going to sit down. I don't think I can walk anymore." She sat on a golf course bench, a total listlessness in her face.

"Darling," she said slowly and in a faraway voice, "we better go and see that doctor in the hotel right away." And after another pause, "I really want to die now."

Panic, helpless panic, shot through me a second time in Sandy's illness, but with Gloria's help, I got her back to the Homestead and called the hospital immediately. This was the time I had overgauged her resilience, I thought. This, finally, was the time that my efforts to give her pleasure and help us both forget the illness were going to end in disaster. What a hell of a place to have it happen!

While Sandy collapsed in bed with blankets over her shivering body, I called the Hot Springs Hospital. On our arrival I had gone into the village on the excuse of buying something. Instead, I had gone to the hospital to meet the people there and talk about the possibility of getting a transfusion started. Since we'd survived trips to New York, Boston, Florida and the Eastern Shore of Maryland with no grave mishaps, I had been lulled into thinking we were safe away from home. So when I had spoken with the nurses and technician about a transfusion for Sandy's anemia, I had done so casually, and they had answered in an equally casual way that they did do transfusions.

Now I spoke with the nurse in charge and told her I wanted to bring my wife in immediately and have blood tests done. The nurse agreed, but when I asked if one of the doctors in practice in the town might be called in to take charge, while I consulted with my wife's hematologist in Washington, she said, "The doctor at the Homestead is the only one here today."

"I'll get in touch with him when we get to the hospital," I answered, "but could you have someone ready to do a hemoglobin and hematocrit as soon as we get there? This is an emergency."

I called a taxi, phoned Arnold Lear in Washington and told him the situation, and said I would call him back as soon as I knew Sandy's blood count.

"Get one of the doctors there to examine her to see if she's had a stroke," Arnold said. But there wasn't any doctor in Hot Springs that day who did neurological examinations regularly.

Once Sandy was in the hospital, I felt somewhat relieved. The technician was gay and pleasant when she was taking a syringe full of blood from Sandy's arm, and we all bantered a bit with relief.

I went back to the lab with her as she tested the blood sample. Her manner changed completely when she read the result. "She only has a hemoglobin of two and a half grams. I've never seen one that low. What kind of anemia *does* she have?"

"It's an anemia secondary to acute granulocytic leukemia," I answered. "I didn't think we would have any trouble down here because my wife just had a transfusion of two pints of blood in Washington the day before yesterday, and her hemoglobin went up to nine grams."

I cut short our conversation because I had to call Dr. Lear again and tell him where we stood. On the phone we spoke about bringing Sandy back to Washington, which was clearly impossible. He decided to give her two bags of packed red blood cells in Hot Springs and spoke with the technician about the details. Only after we hung up did it dawn on us that, of course, there was no blood bank in Hot Springs.

"What do you do about transfusions?" I asked.

"We don't get many transfusions to do here, you know," she answered. "Sometimes we do keep some blood but we use glucose, mostly, until we can transport acute patients to Charlottesville or Washington."

We then called the University of Virginia Hospital at Charlottesville, but their lab didn't have any blood-type A packed cells ready for use. Another phone call, to the regional blood bank in Lynchburg, Virginia, did turn up the blood we needed and the blood bank agreed to send it by air. I had been poring over the skimpy airline schedule in and out of Hot Springs and found that a plane would leave Lynchburg for Hot Springs at 11:15, about a half hour away.

"Let's go back to the Homestead and have lunch," I said, hoping to make all of us feel more comfortable. "We can come back at one and get the transfusion over early in the afternoon."

That operation of calming everyone involved a taxi, a wheelchair, two men to help get Sandy out of the taxi, and about a half-mile walk along the corridors of the hotel with the wheelchair to the freight elevator, the only one that could accommodate the wheelchair. As soon as we sat down to lunch I was called to the telephone. It was the lab technician at the hospital.

"They didn't get the blood to the plane on time. It's back at the blood bank in Lynchburg."

I knew from my study of the schedule that there wasn't another plane until the next day. I had already tried to charter a plane and found it would take a number of hours to make all the arrangements, and since planes flew in the Blue Ridge Mountains only during daylight, it might be morning before one could get from Lynchburg to Hot Springs. I asked the technician if there was any other possible way of getting the blood that afternoon.

"A Red Cross truck could bring it up, but you would have to have her doctor certify that it's an emergency," she said.

At this point Sandy's face was as white as her pillow, her pulse rate was 110, and she had never been so weak. So I called Dr. Lear in Washington again, and he then called both Hot Springs and Lynchburg to confirm that this was an emergency, a true life-or-death emergency. Then we waited.

The technician at the hospital called. "The Red Cross truck can't come up this afternoon," she said. "But everything will be all right. The State Police have already started off with the blood. It should be here in four hours."

The distance from Lynchburg to Hot Springs is 120 miles through curving mountainous roads, but by the time we had made all arrangements at the hotel, gotten Russell changed and Sandy settled into a bed at the hospital, the police car drove up. What a sight! Russell and Gloria were playing peekaboo on the little outside porch of the hospital as the troopers, ornate pistol grips and belt buckles gleaming in the sunshine, stepped out of their dusty brown patrol car, carrying the blood. They had made the trip in just two and a half hours. After great thanks to the highway patrolmen, I hurried into Sandy's room with the genial doctor from the hotel.

Transfusions were used rarely at that small hospital and we all looked around at each other uncertainly after contemplating the various valves and incredibly precious blood in the compressible plastic bags we now had.

The nurse and I did get the plugs in the right places of the first transfusion bag, and I stuck Sandy's vein accurately. The blood started to flow into her, and we took a moment to sigh with relief. Then we had to get back to work. Over the phone Arnold Lear cautioned me about the problem of pulmonary edema, about the dangers of an air bubble in the tubing which could result in an embolism, and about the possibility that there were pyrogens, chemicals that cause fever, in the blood. Fortunately, we didn't even think of hepatitis; the rest of the worries were enough to keep us frightened. His instructions for dealing with any of the complications were simple: "Stop the transfusion." But stopping the transfusion might also mean stopping life, so there was small comfort to be had from any quarter.

There wasn't much to say in the darkened room as the blood dripped slowly into Sandy's vein. I droned on about what we might do that evening, but she wasn't much interested in the future. When I reminisced about the race of the patrolmen to get the blood from Lynchburg to Hot Springs, she perked up and listened more attentively. She was quite intrigued to hear about my conversation with the troopers and the arrangements made to get the blood so quickly.

"You must send a large donation to their welfare fund, and I'll write a note to them when I'm stronger," she said.

She dozed a bit; we took her temperature every half hour; she watched the blood drip, drip, drip into her veins and found it difficult to become comfortable. But mainly, she composed herself, and waited until the end of an unpleasant experience. I was exhausted by this time, and for me, the room had more ominous associations. I wondered how we had ever ended up in the tiny Hot Springs, Virginia, Hospital. Would this be the end of everything? How could Sandy ever get through this, and how could I get her back to Washington?

Sitting in the white hospital chair, with its little rounded metal seat, I half dozed as I held her hand and wondered whether I had the right to subject her to dangers and exhaustion of this kind. Was I merely feeding my wish to turn away from the powerful reality of her death, my personal sense of failure in not being able to help her more? Was I offering her circuses when what was needed was the composure to accept inevitability? I wondered if the efforts we had made about the Eastern Shore of Maryland, New York, Boston, parties in Washington were worthwhile, as she lay there almost immobile, and I was sick with tense fatigue. I wondered whether I was lying not only to Sandy about her illness, but to myself. Maybe I was involved in a totally selfish effort to turn away from despair and the experience all humans face unless they die quickly on some deserted road, careering around the corner in a blue Buick convertible, to be smashed quickly against a sturdy tree. All of my efforts to have her live and die with grandeur were directed toward a certain moment, and then nothing would be left anyway.

Sandy's death was incomprehensible to me, and I began then for the first time to think that the ultimate hurt might come from me, that I would be the one to cause her death by having helped her come to Hot Springs. What an irony, what craziness.

Still, thinking this and watching the blood drip in her arm, I knew she was feeling better because she became quite impatient at seeing the blood go so slowly.

"Darling, why not just speed it up so we can get this whole thing done and get back to the hotel?" she asked. When I left the room for a few minutes, Sandy called me back by clanging her bell. She had noticed that the first bag was almost empty. Like all patients having transfusions, she feared that the next infusion in her bloodstream might be air. We started to give her the second bag of blood, screwing it into the plastic tube, hoping the needle wouldn't dislodge from her vein. Just as we got it started, I looked up at the bag and saw it was marked *B*. We had typed and cross-matched blood from the first bag but had not felt it necessary to do so with the second.

"My God," I thought, "this is type B blood. The whole bag will clot in her!" I quickly closed down the valve and made the blood run as slowly as possible.

"Why are you doing that?" Sandy asked. "I want to get this foolish thing over with."

"You have a little fever. I think you should have some glucose before you get the second bag of blood."

"But I want to get it over with. I don't care about a little bit of fever, and you can give me another antihistamine tablet." I got angry out of panic.

"We're going to change to glucose," I said, running out of the room to get a bottle and to tell the technician the problem. I told her to call Lynchburg and check, and also to check on the receipts she had gotten with the blood. She thought I was being an alarmist and came in to look at the bag. When she saw the *B* on it she hurriedly brought the glucose. As we put the bottle on I jiggled the plastic tube going into Sandy's arm.

"Can't you do it any better?" she complained.

"I'm doing the best I can," I snapped.

Since we had cut the flow of blood to such a slow drip, I was afraid it had clotted and that either nothing had been going in or else clotted platelets had been going in which could form emboli in Sandy's bloodstream. However, the glucose was started and momentarily we forgot that worry as we puzzled over what in the world had happened.

I called Arnold Lear again. The technician

called Lynchburg. The second bag was definitely marked differently from the first. The people in Lynchburg were as puzzled as we were, and Arnold ordered that Sandy should not get any more blood until we could be absolutely certain.

When the technician typed and cross-matched the second bag she found it was A positive. The *B* evidently signified only that it was the second bag. I took a long breath and said, "Let's go ahead." As we started it I thought, " — and I'm responsible for the consequences."

At that moment the hotel doctor returned. I told him about our panicked quandary but he didn't seem to understand or care very much. He sat down beside Sandy and said with a laugh, "Well, everything will be all right. These new blood bags aren't nearly as good as the old bottles we used to have. I remember when I was at the university, we didn't even have blood. We used to give patients dextran." He began to talk to Sandy about patients he had seen at Hot Springs, famous ones, sick ones, odd ones. He and Sandy got into a deep conversation about mutual friends in Hot Springs, the healing value of the mineral waters and other critical questions during the time that I was frantically wondering if I had killed my wife.

The blood was compatible. Sandy had a slight

febrile reaction, but as the second bag gradually dripped into her arm, she became noticeably flushed and more cheerful. It took a long time and she had to lie there throughout the afternoon. Her very complaining about it was comforting. She was alive.

I went back to the Homestead to see how Russell and Gloria were doing. They were playing happily on the grass. I called Arnold one last time and then went back to Sandy. When the second transfusion was finished, she looked crossly at me and the technician as if we were dolts, got up from bed, and put on her blouse. She thanked everyone graciously and began to walk out to the car. The hospital staff stood, amazed, as Sandy, who had arrived in a wheelchair, almost dead and with only $2\frac{1}{2}$ grams of hemoglobin, walked out confidently, smiling, and with "thank you's" to everyone.

At the Homestead, almost recovered myself, I gently suggested a quiet evening in our room with dinner brought in and some reading in bed, but Sandy insisted on going down to the dining room.

"I've given you a bad time of it, we must celebrate tonight. I feel just fine." So she put on a lovely long green dress and walked down to the dinner table.

"Good evening, Mrs. Werkman. You look very

well tonight," Mr. Duncan, the headwaiter, said as he stood behind her chair.

"Thank you," said Sandy. "I had a transfusion this afternoon and it worked wonders for me." She said this as casually as she might have spoken of the healing effects of the sulphur baths, and then asked him what he would recommend from the kitchen.

We had a bottle of champagne with dinner and Sandy said she wanted to dance. As we embraced each other, dancing in the Italian way to a slow, dreamy tune, we murmured to each other about love, and later at the table we chuckled about how we had outwitted Arnold Lear, who had not wanted Sandy to go to Hot Springs at all.

The end of that day was so characteristic of Sandy. She stored away pleasant memories and discarded the rest. Ruefulness, complaint were foreign to her nature. Sleep that night in the high mountains of Virginia was gentle and happy.

Chapter 16

Three days later our plane lifted off the runway of the Hot Springs airport and gently headed us above the scrub pine of the Virginia hillsides toward Washington. The cool, fresh-smelling mountain air, swimming, and hours of gazing toward the blue sky gave Sandy new strength and confirmed my belief in the magical restoring qualities of a spa. Because of Hot Springs we were both able to savor the Washington springtime with pleasure.

Sandy was busy with the publicity and teas before the opening night of the Washington Opera Society's world premiere of *Bomarzo*, a brilliant opera by Alberto Ginastera. She continued her swimming proudly and took Russell to outdoor birthday parties in Montrose Park. I was busy with patients and teaching at Children's Hospital, and both of us became backgammon enthusiasts during quiet evenings at home or during long, deliciously expansive weekends in Maryland.

We had long Saturday lunches outside in our garden, shielded from the warm spring sun by our large maple trees. After cold ham and salami, crusty, soft French bread and a salad, Brie and white wine, Sandy would suggest a walk with Russell to Montrose Park or to Rose Park, a tiny enclave several blocks from our house where children played on swings and dogs got their exercise while their masters watched for the arrival of the police, signaling the need to attach leashes hurriedly. I would plump Russell in his carriage and off we would journey through our black and brass garden door with its gracefully fluted top onto the hot brick sidewalk of N Street. We would guide Russell up and down curbs, tarred streets and the uneven brick sidewalks past the Francis Scott Key Bookshop, then back to the burgeoning crowds of people that were beginning to transform Wisconsin Avenue into a second, clogged Greenwich Village MacDougal Street, and finally, up the hill to the quiet of green Montrose Park, dominating all of Georgetown like a baron's castle.

It was a placid time and Sandy was pleased that her doctors were decreasing her dosage of Prednisone and methotrexate. Her appointment book records:

Off 4 more pills. Hurray.

She was unaware that this decrease signaled a sad resignation to the disease — the pills were simply no longer effective. Worse, the pills were now actively hostile to the formation of blood cells and lowered her resistance to infection. But she saw the reduction in the number she swallowed as a triumph and gloated over each change as a fat person does over a lowering of the pointer on his bathroom scale.

And leukemia continued to insert itself into more of her body. Along with notes in her appointment book about swimming dates and rector's committee meetings at St. John's Church, terse phrases such as "sudden pain in evening," "feeling better, then weak in middle of day," and "bad night" crept in. At first, the pains were small, fleeting backaches, then irritating ulcers, and then they became worse. I wrote her brother James Colt in Boston about the plight we lived with:

I really don't know where we are with Sandy's illness. She has come through a dangerous hospitalization feeling fine. Two weeks ago, when she had a fever of 104°, no blood clotting mechanism and no effective white blood cells to combat infection, I felt as low as I ever have in my life. The next night though, she beat me at gin rummy! She pulled through on magnificent spirit and with the help and devotion of great doctors.

Her trouble now is in the form of many skin infections, like small boils. They are the result of lack of effective resistance to combat even minor infections. Her doctors don't want to start antibiotics again because those drugs upset her already artificially maintained body metabolism. For example, she goes to the hospital next Wednesday for what, in ordinary times, should be a decidedly minor operation for the removal of a small, probably benign, growth. The doctors want to be sure that they don't obscure a low-grade systemic infection, one that would contraindicate such surgery, by giving her prophylactic antibiotics. So, as you can well appreciate, any small intervention brings up the specter of uncontrolled bleeding or bloodstream infection.

I often feel as though we are in a jet plane that has lost its control mechanism, careening through empty high air. I am also acutely aware that time has run out on the percentages. I thought you and your family should know this because, as our happy life goes on day by day, there is little hint of this dark side. Sandy continues to be extraordinarily strong and full of good spirits. Russell is in great shape. With God's grace we will see you at the Cape this summer.

Lisa Colt, Sandy's sister-in-law, read the letter and wrote back:

Jimmy came over tonight to show Harry and me your letter to him. Your ache must be almost beyond bearing, and oh, dear God, how brave you both are. That lovely, poised, utterly dignified and gentle creature that you married seems to have quietly grown up and out in every direction in her capacity to love, in compassion and perception and warmth, and in the delicious, ripe contentment of being loved. And since there has *got* to be beauty or goodness in every single thing that happens in life, it is at least a happy thought that Sandy has grown into a maturity and fulfillment that not so very many people in the world can ever hope to know.

In this twilight time one last delightful event captured our attention, the birthday party Sandy had begun planning back in January on the beach in Florida. She rattled on about Japanese lanterns and arrangements for the orchestra. "I wonder if we can take a chance and have it outside in the garden, or should we take the furniture out of the dining room and have the dancing there?"

Rather sourly, I complained about the expense and effort that would have to go into such an undertaking, but Sandy wagged her finger at me in mock crossness. "I'll do all the arranging and you said the rent money from the Twenty-eighth Street house was mine to do anything I want with. A party for you is what I want to do with it."

I remembered the last time she had stood firm on the "the rent money is mine to do anything I want with." At Christmas she had surprised me with the complete ten-volume hardbound set of Grove's *Dictionary of Music and Musicians*, when I knew that a paperback edition at one-quarter the price was due out in a matter of months. In those moments she made me feel like Eugene O'Neill's penurious father in *Long Day's Journey into Night*, who ranted about the high cost of keeping electric light bulbs burning, and ignored the fact that their light allowed him to see his family.

But more seriously I worried about how much energy the planning of this party would extract from Sandy and about the important possibility that she would not live to see the party. She went ahead, tentatively at first, for I dragged my heels on the idea, trying to divert her thoughts to a more modest celebration. Undaunted, she carried on, and her diary records on various days: "tent man," "Ridgewell's" (the caterers), "Howard Devron" (orchestra leader), "Copenhaver's" (invitation engravers). At that time I remembered, more than a little ruefully, how a close friend had criticized the marriage of a man in his thirties to a very young girl. He said, "He'll be an old man when she's still young and attractive, and he'll die years before her. It just doesn't make sense." Though he was talking about someone else, he also had me in mind, for he commented repeatedly on the gap of years between his experiences and mine when we talked about college days and New York friends. I felt like asking him to lick his own invitation envelope or buy the champagne as Sandy became increasingly engrossed in planning for the party.

The party evening in late May was surprisingly cool, windy and clear for Washington. The tent, dwarfing all the surrounding fences, flapped smartly and guests arrived through an archway of Japanese lanterns after dinners arranged by Sandy at the houses of various friends. Devron's band played songs like "Mountain Greenery" and "Just One of Those Things" in bright tempos, and Sandy and I stood at the entrance to the tent, greeting clusters of happy friends in black tie and long dresses. A few marveled at Sandy's stamina, much less her presence at all, but most came with smiles and pleasure at her recovery, unaware that she had been in bed most of the week and had had a transfusion three days before.

At midnight the band played a chord and Sandy made a very pretty toast, looking most beguilingly innocent, when she wanted to appear most worldly-wise. The band followed with "Happy Birthday" as Gloria, on cue from Sandy, ceremoniously marched in with a large vanilla birthday cake aflicker with a great many candles. We all danced and were very gay, young and old, and the party continued at a peak until 2 A.M. Sandy danced happily and bustled about the entire evening, steering people to the steak tartare and away from the bar to the dance floor. She slipped off to bed a bit early, but a small group of carousing friends joined me in the dining room to sing opera favorites such as "Là ci darem la mano" and "Voi che sapete" in loud, champagne-tuned voices.

It was a perfect evening, and, as I climbed the stairs to our bedroom, pulling at my bow tie and unfastening the studs in my sweat-drenched shirt, I didn't think of the past or the future. That's the way perfect evenings are. I carried in my hand a present Sandy had slipped me during the evening, a handsome set of gold cuff links engraved with A.C.–S.W. With the cuff links was a card saying:

> *Happiest of birthdays to my darling Sidney.*
> *Bless the day you were born!*
> *from*
> *his Alessandra*

I slipped into bed beside her, and for once, didn't stay awake long enough to pray that she would get better.

Chapter 17

At 4 A.M., the darkness of our bedroom occasionally parted by a subdued flash of light from a passing car on N Street, Sandy began to murmur about an aching sensation in her spine. A few moments later, while I was still groggy with sleep and champagne, she called out sharply, "Darling, my back is just terrible. Do something about it." She began to writhe in bed, pain clutching at her back, making sweat form on her forehead and roll down her face.

Her pain was so intense and her voice so unusually imploring that I knew something had changed, something that a pain-killer given by mouth would not control. For the first time I called Dr. Lear in the middle of the night. I was panicked, for I sensed that this was the beginning of the last phase. I apologized to Arnold for waking him up, but he graciously turned my words aside and said he would come over if it would help. Finally, he decided on starting the use of intramuscular injections of opium, Dilaudid in this case.

Hot-eyed and sweaty from champagne, fear, and the peculiar feeling of being flushed and dirty that one has when up again after too little sleep, I kissed Sandy and assured her, unnecessarily, that I would be back soon. "Hurry!" she answered. I pulled on some clothes and raced out of the house, through the squeaking garden gate, to the all-night People's Drugstore on Wisconsin Avenue three blocks away.

It took a bit of discussion to get the prescription filled, as I did not have a special license for prescribing narcotics with me, but the pharmacist, as all other pharmacists during Sandy's illness, was understanding when he heard what the problem was. I had to wait around a bit for him to call in to be sure my license was in order, and to while away the time under the glare of the fluorescent lights, I fussed with hammers and vises on the hardware counter, wondering whether this was the end.

As I padded back home under the arched, still-leaved maple trees, each step resounded on the bricks of the sidewalk in the quiet of the night and the stillness was heightened by the soft buzz of mercury street lights, the churning of air-conditioners and the occasional coughs of homosexuals still standing and hoping for pickups as they waited against the wall of Christ Church.

I ran up the steps to our bedroom. "Here I am, your friendly dope pusher," I exclaimed airily, but Sandy ignored the attempt at humor.

"Hurry with the medicine, it really hurts," she called out.

So at 5:15 A.M. on May Twenty-seventh, I filled the syringe with 5 cc. of sterile water, added it to the powdered Dilaudid in a spoon, mixed the two together, drew the combination into the syringe, chose a place on Sandy's left forearm, swabbed the place with an alcohol swab, and plunged the needle in. I withdrew the syringe plunger a bit. No blood. So, squish, in it went, 30 milligrams of Dilaudid. In a testy voice, Sandy complained, "Don't put it in so fast. It burns like sixty."

I finished the injection and wiped Sandy's arm with the alcohol swab again. She then turned on her other side to protect her back, which pained her so, and in a few minutes fell into a drugged sleep.

I climbed into the other side of the bed and lay there, still sweaty and knotted with the tension of having changed so abruptly from being a lover and adoring husband to being a doctor and bearer of pain, even though it was pain in the service of helping.

Some moments are beyond the reach of ordinary feelings and the confines of usual language. Almost bestial in their rough directness, they are difficult to face and master. This was such a moment, and it reminded me of another time, when as a second-year medical student I had learned to draw blood from the vein of another person. That other person was a close friend, to make the pain more difficult.

One morning of our second year in medical school we appeared in clinical pathology lab, where we learned how to boil urine to look for albumin and how to peer through microscopes at a great variety of blood cells and bacteria. On that particular morning we learned how to draw blood from a patient's arm into a syringe, technically, to perform a venipuncture. The instructions were clear; the only difficult question was who was going to stick whom first. We tossed a coin and I won, or lost, depending upon how one views having to inflict pain on a friend. Following the instructions, I knotted a hollow rubber tube around my friend's upper arm, watched the antecubital veins of the inner aspect of his elbow rise up engorged with blood, and then plunged in with a sharp needle, trying to find the center of a vein in order to withdraw blood for tests. I say plunged, but the actual activity was a slow, hesitant muddling around in tissue, nerve endings and muscle as I sweated and searched for the vein in a frightened, inept way. He didn't help by saying, "Come on. Find the foolish vein and get it over with."

So it was with Sandy. A part of innocence, a part that remains intact in most people who are not doctors or who haven't killed or lived in a hospital or in a jail, was over on that day in medical school, and a further part was torn away in giving Sandy that first shot. Afterwards, sometimes I gave her six injections a day to produce relief from pain. But I knew that once we started on injections, the road would become increasingly dangerous and a point would come when increasing doses of medicine would be necessary, and finally a time would come when she simply no longer existed.

Russell woke up in the early dawn and had to be covered and tucked in before I could fall back into a sleep. Then a second injection to Sandy, in the other arm this time. And some sleep for both of us. But precisely at 8 A.M., unheard of for Ridgewell's, their men, full of gay Italian *buon giorno*'s, came to get the gold chairs and champagne glasses.

175

I knew the tent men would follow, and indeed, they did, creaking the garden gate and apologizing to me as I greeted them in my pajamas, hot and very red-eyed. "The boss didn't think we would need the tent till Monday, but an extra wedding just came up —" Sleep was impossible so I set about emptying ashtrays and putting champagne bottles in their heavy cardboard cartons.

One welcome creaking of the garden gate occurred. A friend appeared clutching a bunch of glorious red roses in his hand, and looking very fresh for 9 A.M. He said, "You and Sandy gave us such a happy time last night. Mary wanted you to have these." I thanked him and he asked, "Where is Sandy?" Then, "She must be tired after all that gaiety last night." I told him she wasn't feeling particularly well and was going to rest in bed for the morning.

This man, who had lost a ten-year-old daughter to leukemia, replied, innocently, "Very sensible of her. Give her our love. Now, both of you be sure to come and play tennis as soon as she's feeling better." And off he went down N Street, leaving more brightness from his brief presence and thoughtfulness than we had from the whole ensuing Saturday of surprisingly clear sunlight.

Chapter 18

 At a certain point in the treatment of leukemia all further moves are blocked. The patient's body becomes the helpless host to a bewildering variety of unwelcome elements, each working against the other, but all toward the common purpose of death. Because so many white blood cells are present in the bone marrow, no room is left for the formation of red blood cells and platelets. Tiny platelets, like millions of Band-Aids, are necessary for clotting to occur. Without them the smallest nick or scratch may bleed endlessly; eventually, too, the blood vessels, weakened by the general disease, rupture and have no means of repairing themselves. The red blood cells, which act as storage containers for oxygen, are too few. Breathing becomes more difficult; parts of the body that need oxygen are starved for it and die, just as a tree dies without water. Even before the whole body dies, the liver, a kidney, the retina of the eye — almost any organ — may become devastated by the lack of air. And all the white cells do no good, for they are sick, crazy, nonfunctioning. Instead of helping to eat up bacteria and other debris in the body, their usual task, they simply float around, clogging and choking blood vessels and gathering together in weedy encroachments as leukemic infiltrations. The usual immune mechanisms of the body are dependent on the white blood cells and they, too, are defunct. Transfusions are artificial ways of replacing red blood cells and platelets. But too many transfusions further depress the bone marrow and the formation of blood and cut off the one small way in which new and somewhat healthy blood cells might be formed. Transfusion reactions at any moment can be lethal, and it is impossible to transfuse a person with blood day after day.

Since the body's natural mechanisms of resistance to infection are inoperative, leukemia patients must depend upon antibiotics for any hope of preventing overwhelming bacterial onslaughts. We had gone through almost all the antibiotics. We could not use the one remaining, as that drug itself may kill red blood cells. But all antibiotics, eventually, lose their strength and new ones had to be tried constantly. Even when the antibiotics are working they pose a special risk of masking a developing infection. The antileukemic drugs — 6-mercaptopurine and methotrexate — kill the unruly white blood cells growing in the bone marrow, but they also kill the few healthy white and red blood cells that are attempting to nourish themselves. And these drugs are an *immense* jolt to the entire body.

Finally, each move — antileukemic drugs, transfusions, antibiotics — cancels out the others and no further move is possible. But unlike chess, this game cannot be begun anew; one does not simply resign and start again or mutter a few words under one's breath about playing better in the next round. There is no next round. Instead, a randomness and a chaos ensue in the body. It had not yet begun with Sandy. She continued to scribble down appointments in her diary and organize little tea parties at her bedside. But her spirit could not thwart the development of large, oozing ulcerations of her buttocks, bleeding in her mouth, the development in her arms of great masses of blood where injections were given, and finally, bleeding in her eyes that clouded the world for her. Ultimately, the two worst ogres were pain and weak-

ness. She could not walk to the bathroom un-
assisted and needed help to turn from one side of
her body to the other to relieve the pain.

And the pain of lying upon open wounds, the
pain from leukemic infiltrations in her spinal cord
that made her back feel like a too tightly wound violin string, pain throughout her whole racked body
became her ordinary companion.

Pain is embarrassing to talk about. Doctors on
their rounds in hospitals ask patients how they are
feeling, but then don't listen or else minimize the
feelings with a feeble joke. But all of us, at one
time or another, owe God not only death but a
good measure of pain. Pain should not embarrass,
because it is, after all, merely one of the sensa-
tional phenomena of the human nervous system. It
is an outrage, though not necessarily a penalty, of
the human spirit. Pascal's statement, "The last act
is bloody, however charming the rest of the play
may be," helps put it all in perspective. But how
can that last act be played with majesty?

Many years ago I bought a secondhand copy of
Edna St. Vincent Millay's book of poems *Second
April* to give to a college girl friend. The book
came from someone's library and its bookplate had
the motto *Apprendre à mourir* (To learn to die). At
the time I was far more interested in the lovely

poems from *Second April* than in the curious motto. It is a wise motto and one whose message became increasingly clear. To die well is indeed to have learned to live well.

As Sandy's pain became increasingly a commonplace, we tried all sorts of ways to outwit and forestall it. The best method to achieve some degree of oblivion was the use of drugs. Tablets of morphine, dissolved with sterile water in a little teaspoon, pulled into a syringe and injected into Sandy's arm seemed to quiet the insistent pressure. I knew in the hot, red-eyed morning, as I waited at the People's Drugstore on Wisconsin Avenue for a first prescription for morphine to be filled, that we had begun to travel down a short, one-way street. Heavy doses of narcotics, given too frequently, may result in death by respiratory arrest. Regular use results in addiction and the need for increasing and, finally, impotent doses of the drug.

Drugs, no matter how powerful, are only the beginning of dealing with great pain. Something has to be done with the hectic energy of illness. Sandy read occasionally. Her bed was strewn with papers and the telephone. Appointments for tea and projected visits to friends in Washington were always on the agenda. But conventional activities wore out their usefulness too quickly. She was unable to concentrate enough to read, particularly when the pain was powerful, and visitors became a greater drain than pleasure.

We began to read aloud. There are not many things suitable for reading and listening to when all of your body aches and exquisite hot pain is present in crucial parts of it. We tried short stories and even novels. Hemingway, Katherine Mansfield, Evelyn Waugh — all failed the test. None of them could capture Sandy's attention or even mine. As spring moved toward the humid heat of summer the only reading that either of us could bear was fairy tales. We settled on their simple fantasy when we found that even poetry had too shocking and demanding a message.

Both of us cherished *The Little Prince* the same way certain college girls were carried away by *The Prophet* of Kahlil Gibran. One section of *The Little Prince* repeatedly delighted us as I read it to Sandy in the early evening. By this time morphine was a regular part of life, and under its effect she fell asleep quite early as I read this lulling passage at bedtime: "And at night you will look up at the stars. Where I live everything is so small that I cannot show you where my star is to be found. It is better, like that. My star will be just one of the stars, for you. And so you will love to watch all the stars in the heavens . . . They will all be your friends."

And: "In one of the stars I shall be living. In one of them I shall be laughing. And so it will be as if all the stars were laughing, when you look at the sky at night . . . You — only — you will have stars that can laugh!"

But somehow the complications of the story, the little prince's diverse adventures and his very active, energetic seeking, were too much for Sandy's confined life. Though polite about it, she became preoccupied with pain or the discomfort of her covers if we tried reading very much of *The Little Prince*.

One most difficult Saturday night, after very little dinner, a laborious bath and an equally laborious attempt at getting to the toilet, Sandy tried to settle down to some kind of ease. I started to read from Lawrence Durrell's *Stiff Upper Lip*, laughing in the appropriate places at the statements of Antrobus and Dovebasket, but it was no go. Sandy complained, "Darling, I just can't get the pillows right," and, "The foam pad has slipped." She was unable to follow anything as pleasantly foolish as Durrell.

Racking my brain, I finally hit upon a great solution, *Andersen's Fairy Tales*, after I had first looked at *Grimm's Fairy Tales* and found them too heavy for our need. That Saturday night and many evenings afterwards "The Steadfast Tin Soldier" (a tale my little son loves to hear over and over), "The Little Mermaid," and the perfect story "The Ugly Duckling" beguiled us.

I would start: "It was glorious out in the country. It was summer, and the corn fields were yellow, and the oats were green, the hay had been put up in stacks in the green meadows and the stork went about on his long red legs. . . ."

Sandy and I both fell into enchanted contentment on reading this story that is poetry and transformation and hope. The ugly duckling who had suffered through so many indignities looked despairingly at the water, and we peered with him:

But what was this that he saw in the clear water? He beheld his own image; and, lo! it was no longer a clumsy dark, gray bird, ugly and hateful to look at, but — a swan!

He was very happy, and yet not at all proud. He remembered how he had been persecuted and despised; and now he heard them saying that he was the most beautiful of all birds. Even the eldertree bent its branches straight down to the water before him, and the sun shone warm and mild. His wings rustled, he lifted his slender neck and cried rejoicingly from the depths of his heart:

"I never dreamed it was possible to be so happy when I was the Ugly Duckling."

What a comfort those fanciful, graceful themes were to us. Reading our fairy tales was what reading the Bible must have been in another era; like reciting poetry or falling in love over again. It took us back to childhood, to bodies and lives whole, safe, pure and hopeful.

Finally a time came when my voice no longer could reach the fresh, protected world of imagination that fairy tales offered. It was too much to give medications, plan for nurses, doctors' visits, arrange for Russell's days, and, all the while, watch life pulling away from Sandy. Instead, I simply lay down beside her in bed and we spun out a kind of shared fantasy about the future that was like a fairy tale but, in some ways, even more soothing.

When reading became too difficult for me, we were blessed with other readers, a whole string of expressive-voiced allies — Leslie Glenn, who hurried in from his work in the Episcopal Church to be at Sandy's side when she needed him; Philip Stern, a writer and tennis partner who had shared many happy times with us; Michael Straight, the best man at our wedding and now our neighbor; Alan Barth; and Sandy's father. Each read selections characteristic of his personality and the phase of Sandy's illness; each contributed immensely to her serenity.

Alan Barth had heavy responsibilities as a member of the editorial board of the *Washington Post*, particularly during Sandy's last days, because of the aftermath of the six-day Israeli-Egyptian war. He was able to come mostly on weekends. But he was a special favorite and, when asked, came on Wednesday afternoons and in the evening on his way home, stopping at N Street before driving on to his house in Cleveland Park. Sandy scribbled his name down in her daily diary, noting the time of his arrival as if he were a dancing partner or a "young man come to call."

She had her hair specially combed, put on a fresh nightgown, and asked Gloria to wash her face, which was usually somewhat sweaty from fever, to prepare for Alan. I always left them alone and he sat in the large silk chair, talking and reading to her. After his visits I could see a relaxation of the tension and pain lines in her face. For him more than for anyone else except her father, and for her father she did not need to make such efforts, Sandy wanted to appear well and strong. She tried to measure up to Alan, and he to her. Though Alan had grown children and other cares and far thoughts, his wish to charm Sandy was great and showed itself in many ways and was reflected from him to her.

One Sunday morning Alan was to appear at 10 A.M.; Sandy had experienced her usual night of pain and sweating despite the air-conditioner, couldn't eat, and had great difficulty in moving from one side to the other in bed. Rain fell all Saturday night until early Sunday. Sunday morning, the sun blazed through the wet leaves on N Street and the day became hot, misty and sultry. Sandy poked at her breakfast and asked Gloria to prepare her for Alan. While I rolled a ball back and forth on the floor between Russell, Niccolo and me in the dining room, Gloria dabbed at Sandy with a facecloth and helped her brush her teeth in bed.

As Russell and I played, I heard the banister creak and then heavy, thumping footsteps on the long staircase. Sandy, leaning on Gloria's arm and holding onto the banister with great firmness, was lurching down the steps. I rushed to the bottom of the steps, frightened and partly irritated that she would risk plunging to her death on her own staircase, yet filled with admiration for her. I tried to help but she waved me away.

She asked me to get a chair from the garden and put it on the porch. She dragged herself out the door and sank, exhausted, into it. Again, she asked Gloria to help compose her so she could surprise Alan. By this time, I was fully enlisted in the surprise and beamed along with Sandy. Alan opened the latch on our garden gate, expecting to trudge up to the bedroom. He was a perfect foil for Sandy's surprise. The happy wonder on his furrowed, freckled face and his delighted "Now, what is this?" were payment enough for Sandy's immense effort. He came up the steps, blushed, and gave her a kiss on the cheek. In place of a reading session, we sat outside and had coffee. Alan was uncertain, wondering whether Sandy had made a remarkable recovery or whether this was some hoax. After a short stay, he left and Sandy asked to be taken upstairs again. She had wanted to spare him the sight of the effort involved in getting back to bed.

On most of his visits, Alan read from Winston Churchill or a contemporary novel, but I think content meant little to both of them. They understood each other, Alan with his infinite kindness and Sandy with her innate desire to please. Alan always stopped to talk with me on the porch for a few moments before leaving.

"How is she, really, Sidney?" he would say.

I told him she had no resistance to infection and

that the ulcers on her buttocks simply wouldn't heal. "Even so, she takes two baths a day and has an ointment put on the ulcers regularly." Alan would touch his hand to my shoulder and leave with a gloomy face.

All the readers contributed their own special focus to Sandy's life, a variety and originality that brightened very long hours. Because of them Sandy had something to look forward to each day and, despite her losing battle, she continued her struggle in good spirits and with some degree of peace.

Chapter 19

 Each night of her life, after brushing her teeth, Sandy pulled at her hair, tilting her head first to one side and then the other, doing at least fifty strokes with a Kent brush guaranteed — not by Kent but by some distant nursemaid or boarding school classmate — to clear the tugs out of a young girl's hair and keep it sleek. Then she applied pink cream and, finally, washed her face in cold water, so she could come to bed fresh and clear. She took off her gray silk kimono — having changed from a wool one months earlier because of the heat — and draped it over the large puffy silk chair nearby and slid into bed. The process, though muted and made increasingly laborious by illness, continued through the warm June darkness. The air-conditioner churned its monotonous rhythm in the background as we kissed each other a "Good night, darling" and turned over to sleep fitfully with bodies touching. Her body was always warm now, and had been for months because of the degree or two of fever that flushed her constantly.

At a moment when, on previous nights, she might have wakened to my kisses by artlessly lifting her hands over her head so I could slither her silky nightgown off, we now merely lay together, fingers entwined, and talked.

Sandy squirmed around, trying to find a comfortable place for her behind. "Ouch! It just hurts all the time. I can't find a single spot in this foolish bed where my back isn't pushed at by lumps. It's like a bed of hot coals. Godfrey's Tweezers, when will this stop?"

"I'll rub your back," I said.

"Never mind. That makes it hurt more. Can't you ask the doctor again if he can think of anything? I don't understand it. I've done all the exercises for my back every day."

"Maybe it will get better when we go to North Haven and you can swim in the ocean," I improvised, for we had talked of flying to Maine for the Fourth of July. We murmured other lulling thoughts and then slept again.

Sandy woke up in the middle of the night when

all outside was quiet except for the occasional screams of teen-agers and the gunning of cars heading home from the nightclubs on the M Street "strip." She was sobbing wordlessly. I took her in my arms, thinking she was having a great deal of pain.

"Darling, darling," I crooned, "it will be all right soon." She continued to cry, and all my questions brought no answers. Finally, I said, "I'll call Arnold or Buddy."

"Don't do that. It's not that."

"Then what is it?"

No answer. Her pitiable crying was like the uncomprehending, inconsolable crying of a child, or of someone being tortured in the next room with the door hopelessly barred to you. I was beside myself and tried to think of any possible thing I could say or do.

In desperation, in the darkness and grogginess of the night, I uttered the unspeakable question always lurking in my brain: "Are you afraid you won't get well?"

"No, Sidney, you know it isn't that."

I wasn't sure she had understood.

"Are you afraid you will die?"

In a clear, strong voice she replied: "I'm not

afraid to *die.*" She emphasized the last word forcefully, almost with contempt.

What was it then? Was she crying over the loss of her clean beauty, now changed to puffy and blotchy horror? Was it the thought of our little son, whom she could no longer mother? Was it because of me? Or was it all the pain and trial, her bright hope and the effort it had cost her mixed together wordlessly in tears?

I was not destined to know; there was just the truth of her one statement: "I'm not afraid to *die.*"

Had she known all the time, then, that she was going to die? The question, worded in that way, is simply too narrow to deal with the complex web of issues involved with knowledge.

Of course Sandy understood in a certain way that her illness was serious; she knew that people die from disease. I had been with her when she heard of the death of treasured relatives. When my mother was near death and Sandy was far away she wrote, characteristically, not of the sadness of death but of the possibility of life: "What a very searching time this is for you in thoughts about your mother's illness and life and death. Death can be comforting and welcoming, and even beautiful when it must happen. All the strength mothers give to their unborn and born is ours to give back to them — and I am sure you are doing this so fully for your mother now."

When I announced the information about the "anemia" to her, she must have made a lightning, instinctive decision to shut off further discussion, probably to shield me even more than herself from the horror of talk whose intent was too clear to people who knew each other as well as we did.

Sandy knew, when transfusions and medicines and wheelchairs invaded her realm of experience, that they were not ordinary accompaniments to a cold or flu or an upset stomach; she was no fool.

At still other times, when life was fulfilling and grand, she must have stretched herself gloriously and closed her ears and mind to the certainty that hovered around her, aware with T. S. Eliot that "human kind cannot bear very much reality."

Medicines, like dreams or alcohol, can alter judgment, ease anxiety, and Sandy was dosed with powerful narcotics for more than a month, and with Prednisone, a hormonal drug that alters mood, during all the span of her illness. These medicines may have affected her attitude toward her illness, though I am not certain they did.

We all recognize somewhere in our thinking, in our nightmares or wishes, that we will die, yet most of us clutch stubbornly at life, able neither to overcome the issue nor to banish it. What I am trying to set out here, and in this entire memoir, is that Sandy, primarily because of her own character, but also because of the help and love of doctors, friends and relatives during this time, scarcely needed to consider whether she would die. She accepted life, exulted in it when she could, and refused to take the time to lament pain and loss. Perhaps this attitude exacted a high price from her and others at some moments, but haven't noble qualities always been rather rare and precious?

Chapter 20

 The trail that for many months had been dramatic, pathetically hopeful, and even made amusing by Sandy's devoted entourage of doctors, relatives, readers and friends, was coming to an end. Our house was now a hospital, complete with rows of medicine bottles, a large supply of syringes and cotton balls, blood stains on the linen and floors and the antiseptic smell of alcohol everywhere. I moved out of our bedroom to a cot in my basement study because Sandy was very restless and in need of constant care. Increasing shifts of nurses hovered over Sandy, dabbing her dry lips with glycerine, putting salves on her sores. I set up a walkie-talkie sound system throughout the house, so I could hear both Sandy and Russell at any time.

The climate of tension and suspense was increased by the external drama of the six-day Arab-Israeli war, which coincided with our own personal struggle.

The Washington weather remained persistently hot. Every trip to Morgan's Pharmacy for more cotton balls, to the Professional Arts Pharmacy for the yellow-brown, sulphurous ointment prescribed by Sandy's surgeon, Dr. Neville Connolly, for the ulcers on Sandy's back and buttocks was like an excursion into the streets of Calcutta. I returned covered with sweat and the peculiar dirty feeling of Washington's sticky humidity. The wilting spiritless leaves outside Sandy's room told the story of heat, as did the dripping air-conditioners sticking out from each house on N Street like perpetual window cleaners perched, backside out, on the facades of the houses. All of our talk and treatment and waiting inside Sandy's bedroom was accompanied by the rhythmic, deep, bass buzzing whine of the air-conditioner.

Troubles increased and stymied us at every turn. It was like a maze experiment in which the rat, though trying all kinds of alternative paths, never is permitted to gain the cheese. We could not fall back on Zen, which teaches that the very act of

197

giving up allows one serenity. We had to continue
on our way. But we still had much to learn on the
trail.

Dr. Connolly came around often to examine the
ulcerations that broke out over Sandy's body. He
usually came late in the evening, carrying a bunch
of roses from his garden in his hand, and was most
professional, excluding me from the room during
the examination, and then calling me in to suggest
a change to cornstarch showers twice a day, the
use of Betadine Scrub, a strong surgeon's soap, to
check infection of the skin, and the continued use
of his special sulphur ointment on the wounds.

Because we had no shower on the second floor
of the house, I hooked up a feeble arrangement of
rubber tubes with garden hose connectors that allowed Sandy to have a makeshift shower without
having to walk all the way to the basement. She
took the two showers a day with religious preci-
sion, surviving breaks in the hose connections that
sprayed erratic jets of water over her and me and
the entire bathroom in a pitiable comedy.

Helping her to the shower was extremely difficult, as she had little strength left in her legs. One
afternoon I was trying to lift her out of bed and
support her on my shoulder to get her to the bathroom. As I pulled her legs around from the bed

to the floor, my elbow hit her squarely in the left eye, raising a big, ugly swelling all around her eye.

Worn out from exertion, and with my now frequent complex of hopelessness–frustration–be pleasant–will nothing work? overwhelming me, I sat her on the bed, then paced back and forth.

"Oh, God, I'm so sorry. I just want to jump out of the window. I might as well kill myself if I can't do anything right. All I want to do in this world is help you and I just hurt you."

"Don't be so silly," Sandy said. "And get me to the bathroom. I can't just dangle here."

Later that afternoon, after the bleeding into her eye had stopped, Dr. Lear had been consulted about what to do, and she had been propped up in bed more comfortably, she received a visit from John Harper, the rector of our church. As he entered the bedroom, before he could say "Hello," Sandy said gaily, "You see, my husband's been maltreating me."

Though that shiner cleared up, Sandy noticed a clouding of her eyes soon after.

"I can hardly see anything on this side of the bed," she said, pointing to her telephone book, mail and dinner tray spread out before her.

"Am I going blind, or what?" she asked in a frightened voice.

I called Buddy, who said she probably had leukemic infiltrations in the retinas of her eyes, a frequent complication of the disease. He later examined her eyes and confirmed that she was becoming partially blind.

Once again the question of what I should tell her came up. Should I tell her her blindness was a complication of leukemia, or should I make up another story? Both of us were terribly frightened by her blindness, and I was painfully tempted to be candid. Instead I said, "Buddy told me it's because of all the strong medicine you're taking. You don't have enough blood and the medicine makes the blood vessels of your eyes close up too tightly."

"But will it go away?"

"Just as soon as we can cut down on the medicine it will begin to clear up," I said.

Diverted for the moment, Sandy turned her attention to stitching on a crewelwork mouse pillow for Ella Burling.

In the evening we drifted into talking of summer and even winter plans. We had hoped to be working in a medical school in Shiraz, Iran, but since that had not been possible, Sandy was eager to move back to Italy, where we had been idyllically happy while I was writing a book. She now encouraged me to write another, and when she had still been able to leave the house, we had gone down to the State Department library together to get some reference material for a book on the psychiatric problems of American families living overseas. She had it all figured out. We would rent a villa in the little village of Arcetri above Florence or on the old road to Siena among the cypresses and stands of maritime pine trees.

Sandy wanted to go in September, saying, "We need time to get settled in and have the whole winter there." Though I knew it was all a hopeless fantasy, I argued that we should wait until January so I could close my work with patients.

"Besides," I said, "the weather will lighten up after New Year's." I reminded her that February is the most glorious possible month in Florence, cold and bright and sunny.

We spoke of going to Cape Cod in the summer and weighed the relative merits of July and August. Sandy wanted to wait until mid-July, reasoning in her lovely, naïve way, "I should be better soon, but I'll need a long time to get my strength back."

One definite plan we made was to spend the Fourth of July weekend with Sandy's brother and sister-in-law in North Haven, Maine. The trip was a real possibility because Phil Stern, who had his own plane, offered to fly us directly to Maine. We weighed the difficulties of flying at night, landing on a private airstrip on North Haven Island, and checking on medical coverage in the area we were going to visit.

But the next day we were back to the multiple problems of pain and weakness again, and thoughts of travel receded. Nothing was working, no new treatment was thought of. We needed a new strategy and called in Dr. John Adams, a fine orthopedist, who came to examine Sandy to see if there was any way to ease the constant pain in her back.

I asked if an X ray of her lower back would help in determining the cause of her pain. He didn't think so. "But X ray . . ." he repeated. "If she has a leukemic infiltration in her vertebrae, possibly a light dose of irradiation will help it."

After much deliberation among various doctors, for X-ray treatment might bring on further complications, it was decided to take Sandy to the George Washington Hospital for several treatments. I borrowed a wheelchair from Children's Hospital. Michael Straight came over from his house across the street, and we picked her up from bed and settled her in the wheelchair. Maneuvering the wheelchair out of the bedroom, Michael in front and I behind, we started down the steep, narrow staircase with Sandy.

All was in readiness. Gloria stood at the bottom of the steps with a coat. My car was double-parked in the street, engine running. We descended the first step easily — too easily — for suddenly we lost control. Sandy and the wheelchair began to lurch down the staircase, with Michael being carried in front of it as if he were impaled and me almost falling over the banister, trying to stop it. It was Sandy, amazingly, who saved us. Instinctively, even in her weakness, she grasped the railing and held on for dear life. We came to a halt in a ludicrous heap.

"Stop it this instant," she said. "I'm going to walk down. We'll all be killed doing it this way." And walk down she did, as Michael and I stood aside meekly. I offered the wheelchair again at the front porch.

"No thanks," she said. "That thing is too dangerous."

She made it to the car on our arms. In the meantime a taxi got stuck behind my double-parked car. The driver started blowing his horn and shouting. A neighbor thought the taxi was pointing out the

Kennedy house to tourists, and began to call out to him to be on his way, and furthermore, never to come back. The gardener at another house across the street thought our neighbor was shouting at him, so he shouted back. During all this we slipped quietly in the car and drove away.

We came home in the early afternoon. "I better get the wheelchair," I said.

"Not on your life!" Sandy said.

Though we trundled her to the X-ray treatment clinic one more time and she was pleased that "something is being done again," the treatments were not really helpful and the effort involved for her was just too great.

The next day, another wet, hot, sticky morning, an ultimate change began to show itself. Sandy woke up in a befogged state. In an overly precise, totally unnatural voice she asked me to bring her bacon, eggs and coffee for breakfast. I fixed breakfast, as Gloria was sleeping, on what was supposed to be a free day for her. Because of her blindness, Sandy couldn't hold her coffee cup straight up, yet she refused my help in getting it to her lips. The coffee spilled and we had to change her nightgown. I prepared a new breakfast, as the first one had gotten cold, and laboriously, Sandy tried to eat again but spilled food a second time. The pain in her back increased, and we had to stop breakfast to shoot another dose of morphine into her.

She asked for breakfast yet again, and I prepared bacon and eggs a third time, but she was unable to concentrate on eating or drinking and fell into a half sleep. Repeatedly she asked for breakfast throughout the day and into the evening, sometimes changing her request, sometimes demanding the same food brought only a few minutes before.

"Please," she said imploringly, "bring me my breakfast. I want tea. This isn't tea. Why do you do this to me?"

When I was worn out, Gloria came upstairs to change Sandy's nightgown and try to get her to eat something. Kneeling at the bedside, Gloria gently brought a cup to Sandy's lips, but the tea spilled again, and despite Gloria's sweet entreaties of "Señora, please have un poco tea, it make you feel better," Sandy brushed the cup away and crossly asked for the very tea she had rejected.

Buddy came that afternoon and we had a long, desperate talk. Several days previously, in conference with Arnold Lear, Ed Adelson and Jack Rheingold, we had decided to cease all treatment. Nothing could be gained, the doctors thought, by any more medication or transfusions. Any further treatment might prolong Sandy's life a short time, but at the cost of much greater pain than even large doses of the strongest narcotics could control. So Sandy just got morphine and vitamins, and she was well aware of the change in the treatment plan, even though she was developing new complications almost daily — difficulty in swallowing, the blindness, swelling of her abdomen.

While Buddy and I were talking, another devoted friend, Larry Kubie, came in. He had been a preeminent psychoanalyst in New York City for many years and had recently retired to Towson, Maryland. He had loved Sandy from the moment he met her, in the singular way many older men did. She brought out in them some of their buried youthful thoughts and desires, their simplicity and courtliness, when to most others they presented only their grand, austere, distinguished sides.

After visiting with Sandy briefly, Larry joined Buddy and me in my basement study, where we continued our talk about the future.

"Now, old man," Larry started in his avuncular, concerned way, "you've done everything you can for her. There is nothing more to do. Let her die peacefully."

"But she knows what's happening," I said. "And she's not dying peacefully anyway."

"She really doesn't comprehend," Larry continued. "The amount of morphine she's taking is bound to dull her greatly, even if she seems to be aware of her situation. She really isn't though, you know. I've seen this happen many times. The only decent thing to do now is withhold medication and just give her fluids to keep her comfortable. . . ." He looked to Buddy.

Buddy, ever thoughtful and respectful, agreed in a general way with Larry, and they talked for a bit about blood counts, leukemic infiltrations and Adolf Meyer, the professor of psychiatry at Johns Hopkins, where both of them had trained.

Returning to me, Larry offered many reasons for not prolonging Sandy's pain. Then he spoke of what I would do with Russell after Sandy died, remarking on how fortunate I was to have "the girl," meaning Gloria.

I was relieved, that time, when Larry left, for I was incredulous at his saying that we should "let her die." Though I thanked him for his concern and advice, as soon as he left I turned to Buddy. "Why can't we give her one more transfusion?"

"It just wouldn't help, Sidney," Buddy said wearily and got up to make a phone call.

When we ended our talk in the late afternoon, I still hoped to find some way, perhaps a miraculous way, to redeem the situation. The rain had stopped and Washington was at its most brilliant. The rain had cooled the atmosphere and lifted the humidity and a yellow-orange evening sun was shining through the leaves from a rare blue sky.

Sandy's calls for breakfast finally receded into a haze of weakness and morphine, and she was able to rest comfortably in the early evening. I stayed with her a bit and then left her with a dear, gentle nurse for the long night vigil.

The situation was clearly beyond me, and I turned to Sandy's parents for help. Two months earlier I had received a most helpful letter from Sandy's father, when he was told by his sons the true hopelessness of Sandy's illness. It read:

30 March 1967

Dear and Gallant Sir,

I have had, and have, a good idea of what you have been experiencing in these past few days.

Enough to blow the top of one's head off, I am sure. As I am equally sure that you have conducted yourself like the hero which you are in my book.

I am always available and at your command.

God bless.
H. F. Colt

Now I needed his proffered help, and a brief phone call quickly brought Mr. and Mrs. Colt to

Washington from Hot Springs, where they were spending several weeks.

Sandy's mother was a great help, adding gay flowers throughout the house and buying Russell toys and books. But Mr. Colt was my firm support, for he could reach both Sandy and me with lightness and wit.

He appeared regularly in the morning from a friend's house nearby in Georgetown where he and Mrs. Colt were staying. When Sandy wanted sausage for breakfast and we had run out of it, he would immediately clap on his outlandishly rumpled ten-gallon Texas hat and be out the door toward Scheele's with a comment like "Dear me, dear me. We'll just have to slaughter another hog and send it by air to Wisconsin to get the Jones Dairy Farm to make some sausage for us."

He would return shortly, loaded down not only with sausage, but also with Keiller's marmalade, a carton of Camel cigarettes, a large box of kitchen matches, sweet butter and bottles of Perrier water, for he declared that Washington tap water was "unpotable." He would help prepare Sandy's breakfast and the three of us would sit together in her bedroom a few minutes while he said amiably grumpy things about the Washington morning newspaper, which he continued to call the *Herald*, even though that paper had merged years ago with the *Washington Post*. Doing the *New York Times* crossword puzzle over a cup of coffee in Sandy's bedroom, he would look up at both of us and say, "Now, here's a challenging one for you. What is the Italian word for 'slow,' five letters?"

Several days passed and Sandy's condition continued to deteriorate, as did her spirits. By Monday afternoon, June 26th, we had come to a flat calm. I was no longer able to answer her questions or comfort her very much. My clumsy jokes were greeted by indifference, my attempts to read by sighs of pain and complaints about the smell of the room. Still, I held her hand and tried to say pleasant things, but I barely disguised my hopelessness.

I gave up and trudged down the stairs to the sitting room, where Mr. Colt was still doing the *Times* crossword puzzle.

"What can I do for you, old boy?" he asked, looking up above his glasses and cigarette.

"Would you go up and be with Sandy awhile?" I asked. "She's in a lot of pain."

He jumped up from his chair as if a military alert had sounded, and lumbered up the stairs ahead of me, puffing and grunting, as he approached his favorite daughter's room, where she lay on her bed, crying out in uncontrollable pain.

Here was his last child, a love child, whose life paralleled the brilliant Washington period of his otherwise spotty external career. Her development and maturity had offered the promise of a substantial fulfillment to fantasies that lived within his entire family.

Once, when I was courting Sandy and she was uncertain whether I was a proper person to marry, she told me in her unselfconscious, naïve way, "You know, darling, I'm sort of the star of my family. Everyone else has been stopped by troubles of one kind or another, but I haven't."

Her family is filled with stars, but she was the least complicated or encumbered one. And it was this star, this promise, that her father approached on a deathbed.

His first comment on surveying this distressing scene was "Dear me, dear me. That reminds me of a story." He settled into a chair, grumbled at the hot-water bottle he sat on, and began to tell of being sick as a child on shipboard in the bay of Constantinople. Sandy had heard the story perhaps eighty-five times, but he told it so precisely, so well, and so wittily, that in a few minutes both Sandy and I were entranced and no longer thinking of pain or fear. Mr. Colt looked for a book to read, and as he settled in, I left the room and allowed those two incredibly bound-together spirits to share their strengths and a variety of grace, which is of minimal importance in ordinary life but invaluable in the clutches.

Mr. Colt came away in about a half hour, saying that Sandy was dozing but had asked for help to go to the bathroom. He left her to the nurse and slumped down in his living-room chair, surrounded by his Perrier water, Camels, and the crossword puzzle, as if he were some ineffectual old man sitting in his club. Appearances are deceiving.

In the late afternoon Les Glenn bounced in to read again. He was quite puzzled as to what would be most appropriate for Sandy. I told him she took in little of what was said and that his presence was more important than what he read. He, too, stayed with her about a half hour and returned downstairs. Hesitantly, he asked how she was, but then gave his report before hearing my answer.

"She told me, 'I don't know if I can stand it much longer. They've given up on me, now.' "

Les continued. "I said some prayers with her and we spoke about faith and the far, great strength of faith, but she did a lot of crying, poor dear. How much longer can this go on, Sidney?"

I wondered that too, and was powerfully influenced by the conference I'd had with Buddy and Dr. Kubie. But I simply could not stand to give up on Sandy or have her feel that she was beyond aid.

Philip Stern phoned and asked about reading. I told him she was in terrible shape and couldn't concentrate well enough to listen to reading. He reminded me that he had checked out his airplane and that the pilot stood ready to go to the Cape at any time. We no longer hoped to go to Maine, because of inadequate emergency medical facilities there, so I had conceived the idea of taking Sandy back to Cape Cod. Even though she could no longer see, she would enjoy the sounds of seabirds and the mixed fragrances of bayberry and pine and salt air. When Phil and I spoke about this new plan, he too became quite excited about the idea.

I felt we had to continue to offer something to Sandy, and so I called Buddy about the plan. He was entirely against it, and we had a long, annoying argument. When personal argument failed to sway me, he said, "She has only 4 grams of hemoglobin. She just won't make it up to the Cape, Sidney. And Arnold Lear won't give her any more transfusions. He doesn't think her system can stand it, and besides he said it was simply cruel."

I blew up at this. "What kind of cruelty is greater, letting her feel hopeless or causing a little discomfort getting her in a plane?"

Buddy said he would come over that evening. He said he would have a hemoglobin and hematocrit done the next day and would type and crossmatch her blood in case they changed their minds.

I pointed out to him that Sandy quizzed me regularly about why no more transfusions were being given and why the medication had been stopped.

"Sidney, there's just nothing more that anybody can do," he said. But by the end of our talk, after he had visited with Sandy, he agreed to consider the possibility.

"Let's go down to the airport and look at Phil Stern's plane," he said with new enthusiasm.

"Now?" I asked.

"Of course. Leave Sandy with her nurse and we'll go down and look at it."

I then told Sandy of our Cape Cod plan and she was truly delighted by it. She loved the thought of going back to Wings Neck in a small plane and asked how we could arrange to get her from the airport to her family's house. I told her we would work out those details but first needed to look at Phil Stern's plane. I kissed her good-night, got in Buddy's car, and we drove toward National Airport. In the car Buddy presented further arguments against flying.

"Sidney, suppose she has a hemorrhage in the plane or the plane crashes? Those small planes are dangerous."

"A crash would be just great," I said. "There's nothing I would want more."

"You mean you wouldn't care if she died?"

"I would be so happy to be able to die with her," I said.

"That may be all right for you and Sandy," Buddy replied, his voice becoming quite stern. "But what about Russell? What about Gloria? What about the pilot? Would you want them to die too?"

I had nothing to say. His view of humanity was so much grander than mine that all I could do was touch him on the shoulder and nod my head in stunned agreement with his logic.

Buddy continued to try to dissuade me from the whole idea, but as he described how tough he had been on pilots during World War II when he was a flight surgeon in the Pacific, he became more interested in the positive side of flying, even as he told of grounding injured pilots who wanted to continue to fly, and of sending aces back to the United States. Then he recalled some of his own exploits of doing operations on pitching ships and being reprimanded for starting blood transfusions during perilous airplane flights. He ended by becoming enthusiastic, himself, about the flight to the Cape.

This hot, breathless Washington evening we prowled around small planes until we found Phil Stern's. Peering in it, we figured out a possible way for Sandy to settle in for the trip. But it was not a convenient plane for her, and Buddy suggested that we see about chartering an ambulance plane. We found one that could handle a stretcher, Russell, Gloria, me and the pilot, and contracted for it. Buddy and the pilot, both World War II Air Force veterans, made lots of special private plans between themselves and became immersed in happy reminiscing.

As we drove back along the George Washington Parkway in the dark night dotted by the lights of the lovely bridges arching across the Potomac to Arlington, both of us felt new hope and even a certain lightheartedness.

Tuesday morning the medical student, who came by three times a week to draw blood, was greeted by Sandy's statement that "you won't need to come for a while. We're going to fly up to Cape Cod on Thursday to be with my family."

He was surprised, but he had learned to take in

a great deal without questioning since he had begun drawing blood in our house. On his first day he had been a mere technician doing his job. I had cautioned him that my wife did not know her diagnosis and that he was not to show her the slips from the laboratory tests, for beside the word "Diagnosis" was the clear statement, "Leukemia." Gradually, he was drawn into our family because of Sandy's warmth and graciousness with him. He had a regular cup of coffee with us in her bedroom, stopped to play with Russell and Niccolo for a moment on his way out, and made a special effort to take her blood early in the morning so she could then go on to bathing and having breakfast.

Later in the morning I went to have a conference about the trip with the assembled hematologists. Arnold Lear was strongly opposed to the idea, since Sandy could not be moved to a hospital and it was too dangerous to give a transfusion at home. The others were equally grave and emphasized the concept that one must accept the end when it comes. After leaving that gloomy meeting, I found a ten-dollar parking ticket on my car to boot.

Tuesday afternoon and evening I continued to talk with Sandy about going to the Cape and she, very rationally, said she just didn't have the energy to go unless she had a transfusion. But she mused about the bedroom on the first floor of the house at Wings Neck and how easily it could be made comfortable for her. On Buddy's evening visit he still spoke against the transfusion, but not with great conviction. Then Phil Stern dropped by and the three of us talked together. Phil had gotten clearance for the plane to land at Otis Air Force Base near the Colts' summer house. Harry Colt, Sandy's brother, arranged to have an ambulance come from the volunteer fire department near the Air Force base and transport Sandy to the house. Nurses had been gathered on the Cape, and the Red Cross blood station was alerted to help.

Buddy had final arguments against the plan. "Any move she makes in the plane will be painful. How can she get decent nursing attention in the air?"

I told him I could start a transfusion in the air if needed. As I saw Buddy to his car, he said, "If she can get through tonight, I think we'll do it." What a relief; we had something to look forward to again! I went back to Sandy and told her the good news, leaving out "if she can get through tonight." She asked me to snuggle with her in bed, and I was easily beguiled into taking off my shoes and lying close to her.

We talked a bit about the plane for the Cape and she then said, rather dreamily, "I love you so much. You've been everything, everything to me. Take care of Russell." I caressed her arm and warm cheek and now bloated belly and told her we would get through all this and soon be on the Cape.

"We'll listen to the gulls and Canadian geese and the foghorn at Cleveland's Ledge."

"But they aren't doing anything for me," she said.

"They will. We all will," I said.

On Wednesday there was much discussion between Mr. Colt and Phil Stern about the ambulance plane and Cape Cod. Mr. Colt became a kind of message station and even called up Otis Air Force Base. In his charming way he reported to me, "I just called up the War Department and they don't know anything about a civilian plane being cleared to land at Otis Air Force Base. Typical War Department bungling. Why you might get up there and be blown right out of the sky." I assured him that we would double-check, but he was having fun too.

Sandy's reported hemoglobin on Wednesday was only 2.5 grams. She was listless and depressed as the whole day dragged by. Buddy called several times about the plane and our plans.

At 6:00 P.M. Buddy appeared with a great smile on his face and two bags of packed cells in his hands. He had won over Arnold Lear to the transfusion and the dream of flying to the Cape. We both hurried up to Sandy's room to show her the cells. She was transformed with pleasure and asked to have a large dinner to prepare herself for the transfusion.

Because of her low blood pressure the cells had to be hung quite high, but we had no stand. Harking back to an earlier era in medicine, I got a stepladder, climbed to the top of the curtain rods, and tied a bag of cells to them.

Soon after, the transfusion began. Sandy perked up and took some lemonade. Buddy stayed through the whole first bag and started the second before he went home. He promised to visit us on the Cape, and again, we shared with him our plans to go to Italy in the fall. Sandy had an excellent night. She slept soundly for the first time in many days and awakened rested on Thursday morning.

Thursday morning was full of bustle and sorting of cotton balls, clothing and Russell's diapers. Sandy wanted to pack a favorite blue cashmere sweater because of the cold Cape evenings in June.

We made many phone calls to double-check plans and arrange for my medical coverage in Washington.

In the morning Sandy held court for her mother and father, Gloria, Buddy and me. We shared our high anticipations of the trip and became immersed in happy details of bathroom needs and a search for a movable stretcher on wheels at the Cape so she could lie outside during the day. We even joked about getting the stretcher down the steps of the cliff in front of the Colts' house—" Only until I can walk on my own steam," interjected Sandy — so that she could be close to the lapping sea.

Gloria brought Russell to Sandy's bed for his morning romp there. As Russell played on the bed, sliding along the blue silk blanket cover and pulling at his mother's rubber seat pad, his diapers full of bowel movement, Sandy said mischievously, "I know Russellino's here, because I can smell him." She cradled him on her shoulder and gave him a blind kiss when Gloria put him close to her before taking him back to his nursery.

Those were her last natural words, for she became increasingly listless and still. She ate little in the afternoon and fell into a sleep that no longer seemed animated or human. The special climate of death stole in on the room that afternoon, silent but unmistakable, like a soft, enveloping Cape Cod fog. We canceled plans for the flight and settled in beside her bed and in the living room to compose ourselves and wait for eternity to touch her. She must have had a massive brain hemorrhage sometime during the day.

Chapter 21

On Friday, June 30, 1967, at 8:41 A.M., Sandy's painfully overworked body stopped functioning. All Thursday night she lay in bed, rumpled and hot, breathing heavily and with great effort. Her shoulders moved with her rib cage in giant, grotesque rhythm. You could sense the urgency of her lungs, needing more and more air, because there was so little blood to transport oxygen. To one watching those terrible heaving breaths, Sandy seemed a sailboat tied up at a dock during a storm, lashed and torn by unseen, giant waves that raised her high in the invisible water, seemingly safe, and then crashed her down suddenly as each wave receded, having done its damage. Again and again and again into an infinity of gulping, hopeless breaths.

The heaving, noisily gulping breaths continued all night. The nurse regularly moistened Sandy's lips with glycerine and swabbed her burning cheeks with a cool cloth. The room was eerily dark; a shaded standing lamp faced toward the medicine table and served the nurse as a light for reading. She said, in the simple words of countless nurses to loved ones watching and waiting, "You'd better get some sleep. There'll be a lot to do to-morrow."

At 4 A.M. on that dark night I was awakened by a cracking lightning-and-thunder storm. I closed the windows in the living and dining rooms and then went to Russell's nursery for a moment, where his air-conditioner was whirring away more softly than Sandy's and where his infant's breathing was quiet and soothing to hear. Then to Sandy's room. The nurse was busy over Sandy, smoothing her nightgown and applying ointment to the ulcers on her body, though more from devotion and empty continuity than for any practical reason. The tortured, heavy breathing continued. No real words came and less Dilaudid was needed, but periods of pain returned, when all Sandy said or allowed herself to say was "Ouch, ouch, ouch, OUCH, OUCH, OUCCCHH!" and "Godfrey's Tweezers."

Eight milligrams of morphine helped, but not in any immediate fashion, and it was difficult to know, with Sandy so filled with drugs and with so little functioning brain left, what was Sandy and what was reflex sound from a distant sleep. But even that night, weakened as she was by disease, she raised herself on her elbows and exchanged a hot pillow for a cool one.

At 7:30 A.M. the nurse left, suggesting as she fussed for the last few minutes over Sandy that Mr. and Mrs. Colt not come in that day to see their daughter so ravaged. I stayed with Sandy several minutes, held her black-and-blue arm, and then heard Russell gurgling in his crib. I swooped him up from his sweet, yawning awakening and brought him to his mother for a final kiss, then hurried down the stairs with him to Gloria.

I had to tell her abruptly, "La Señora is close to death." Gloria, only twenty-two, who began with us as a nurse to a new baby in a young and buoyant family, had been caught up, unawares, in disaster. And this was the first time I could share the secret with her.

She blanched, shrieked, and then rushed to the kitchen to cry and through her tears call "No, No, *No*" endlessly, until her friend Elena arrived to help comfort her.

I returned to Sandy and whispered my love in her unhearing ear.

In the hour before the day nurse arrived, I stayed with Sandy, aimless, drifting. Her heavily labored breathing changed to a very quiet, low, very slow regularity just after eight. She was now breathing mainly with her abdominal muscles, no movement of her neck, her sternum or clavicles, just that quietness, even serenity, that I had known would come since October 26th.

After minutes of slow, very, very shallow half breaths, she breathed once, then stopped breathing for fully a half minute, inspired again, stopped, and never breathed again. I put my stethoscope to her so lovely breast and knew her body had died at 8:41 A.M. I held her hand, kissed her lips and cheek, and cuddled her body against mine for the last time.

Chapter 22

Then all the turmoil of death began — a phone call to Buddy Gusack, the writing of an obituary, the gathering of relatives and friends, the chill commercialism of undertakers. And a terrifying moment when Russell, lying in my arms, gulped four deep, consecutive breaths and then stopped breathing. Thank God, he breathed out finally, and never had another episode of breath holding.

But some quiet returned, and two days later, on Sunday, July 2nd, Sandy was borne into St. John's Church.

At our wedding Sandy cared greatly that the correct tune of a hymn, "Oh, Pray for the Peace of Jerusalem," sung at her father's school, be used. At her funeral I cared only that Russell be with me when I had to smile and speak with friends and relatives after the service, and that Mark Thomas play "The Dance of the Blessed Spirits" from Gluck's *Orfeo ed Euridice* on his platinum flute. Mark played that most moving of all themes, the reuniting of Orpheus with his Eurydice in the Elysian fields, the theme that healed the wound of Orpheus's cry, " 'If fate denies us this privilege for my wife, one thing is certain: I do not want to go back either; triumph in the death of two.' And with his words, the music made the pale phantoms weep."

Sandy's ashes were committed to the ground in a low corner of the Oak Hill Cemetery in Georgetown near where we had taken our first walk together and Sandy had wanted to turn left up toward the Massachusetts Avenue Bridge, but I, sensing that she was strong-willed but not infallible, persuaded her to turn right toward the "Q" Street "Buffalo" Bridge and my house. I said these words to our friends gathered in the cemetery:

"Let me share with you something of the last eight months of Sandy's life.

"During those months sleep was taken from her by immense doses of body-shattering medicine, so she left our bed at four in the morning to go to the kitchen and bake delicious bread.

"Though Sandy was a natural and particularly graceful athlete, tennis was denied her by illness — and she was just becoming the fine player she was capable of being — but she regularly swam fifteen lengths of a long pool until two months before her death.

"When she developed severe back pain, her response was to exercise in bed without complaint to strengthen her back muscles. Running and feeling the full freedom of her lithe body were denied her. Yet, even I never heard one word of self-pitying regret.

"Her lovely, slim form and sparkling face were changed to puffiness by cortisone, but after an initial deep breath over the disfigurement — and Sandy had lived her adult life knowing as a mere fact that she was a bewitching creature — she continued to feel beautiful, and to be beautiful. Large blotches of discoloration in her skin, weakness, pain and, finally, blindness overtook her.

"How did all of this affect her? Almost not at all.

"She danced with such delight at our party on the twenty-sixth of May and joked the day before she died, about our infant son Russell as he lay beside her. Her only regret, and it was a great one, was her inability to play vigorously with Russell.

"Not only in illness, but in all of her life that I

shared, she was directed toward making the moment charming, the experience useful, whether in taking Russell regularly to visit my father in his nursing home, making some needlepoint for her own childhood nurse in the last months, encouraging and so enjoying visits from her family and our friends in Washington or the country, or leaving the Peace Corps when she felt her characteristic work was done to look for the next important experience in life, which so fortunately for me was our marriage. Sandy cared, as a beguiling child cares, that she please those around her, and she was fulfilled, with the overflowing totality of a child's fulfillment, by the joy she gave others.

"Old-fashioned compass points — joy, virtue, responsibility, generosity of spirit, pride in her family and, when nothing else remained, elemental valor — defined the boundaries of her life.

"Many people have asked me if she knew the name of her death. And I ask, Does a brave soldier fight less gallantly for knowing the next bullet will enter his body? The question is irrelevant to great lives. And I say, with assurance and some objectivity, that hers was a great life.

"That we are here together at this moment on this ultimate field, as lovers and mourners of Alexandra, blesses our lives. Those who have found their Way need no explanation for this morning.

"Those of us who have not, merely stand in awe of having shared the grace of one of God's spies on this earth. That there are lessons about courage and brilliance of spirit is plain.

"If there is any lesson of comfort in her death to us here still alive, each of us must find it as he can."

Afterword

After Sandy's death a kind of controlled panic seized me, a panic eased slightly by the recognition that I had been witness to an awesome phenomenon — like that of sighting a great passage of immense hawks soundlessly, lazily floating in the clean, big, blue sky above Gray's Peak on the western slope of the Rocky Mountains. In the weeks that followed her funeral a rain of letters arrived. As I read the letters and wept over many of them, I began to appreciate these words from *Antigone*: "Only a little time to please the living, but all eternity to love the dead." And I began to understand something of the meaning of immortality.

Sandy was loved uniquely, and her death merely established a permanence for the place she had made in the lives of those who had known her. Occasional phrases and sentences from some of the letters I received speak of the effect she had on her friends and relatives:

Sandy's example of courage and determination was almost superhuman. She had such a marvelous natural vitality and true goodness. How proud your son will be when he is old enough to understand what a rare person his mother was.

———————

One encounters a person like Sandy rarely in a lifetime, and I suppose the only tenable position at a time like this is to dwell on the privilege of having known her at all — the chance to have been near one superlative human being.

Though doctors gave so much, everything that medicine could offer and their great compassion devise, a single man carried the pivotal burden of making Sandy's final time on this earth bearable. Henry Francis Colt, sometime colonel in the United States Army during the Second World War, able hockey player at Harvard, head boy at his boarding school, whose later accomplishments may seem modest to the outside observer, was the hero — witty and sublime and calming by turns — of his daughter's illness. Perhaps all his life was preparation to play this role, however devastating it was to him.

233

His own words in a letter he wrote after Sandy's death to the Reverend Arthur Lee "Tui" Kinsolving, retired rector of St. James' Episcopal Church in New York City, and an old family friend, transcend any description I could offer of him. This letter is the only utterance Mr. Colt ever allowed himself about the death of a favorite daughter. It was written, not to me nor to his grandson, Russell, for that would have seemed sentimental to him, but in answer to a note from Tui Kinsolving. In the letter, forwarded to me by Tui, Mr. Colt pens his own portrait, and through his words you may see something more of what his daughter was like.

July 28, 1967

Dear Tui,

Thank you for your letter.

I want to say a few things to you particularly.

Sandy and Sidney's married life was the happiest I have ever observed. Each had an industrious, useful, fruitful life of work. And their home was full of good music, good talk, good fun, and lovely friends.

Their conduct in their last terrible six months has been beyond praise. Sandy, under the hottest fire possible, bore her trials with a gallantry and quiet dignity that amazed all observers except this pilgrim. It did other things to me. Sandy never realized that she was fatally ill.

We have had letters about Sandy, scores of letters,

from Great Britain, France, Italy and, of course, this country. Some from people who are unknown to us. I think it may be said of that gallant and radiant spirit that during her brief span on this planet she adorned and illuminated the scene.

Our love to you both.

Henry F. Colt

I have written this memoir of Sandy for Russell, for all those who shared our experiences, and for those who learn of them here; but as I think back now, I am quite certain that, above all, it was for a noble father that it is written.